Global Public Health Vigilance

Routledge Studies in Science, Technology and Society

Global Public Health Vigilance

Creating a World on Alert

Lorna Weir and Eric Mykhalovskiy

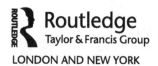

Routledge
Taylor & Francis Group

LONDON AND NEW YORK

First published 2010
by Routledge
2 Park Square, Milton Park, Abingdon, Oxon OX14 4RN

52 Vanderbilt Avenue, New York, NY 10017

Routledge is an imprint of the Taylor & Francis Group, an informa business

First issued in paperback 2012

© 2010 Taylor & Francis

Typeset in Sabon by IBT Global.

Library of Congress Cataloging-in-Publication Data

Weir, Lorna
  Global public health vigilance : creating a world on alert / by Lorna Weir and Eric Mykhalovskiy.
    p. cm. — (Routledge studies in science, technology, and society ; 10)
  Includes bibliographical references and index.
  1. World health. I. Mykhalovskiy, Eric. II. Title.
  RA441.W395 2010
  362.1 — dc22
  2009033868

ISBN13: 978-0-415-95842-4 (hbk)
ISBN13: 978-0-415-81060-9 (pbk)

Contents

Figures and Tables

FIGURES

TABLE

Abbreviations

BSE	Bovine Spongiform Encephalopathy
CDC	Centers for Disease Control and Prevention (USA)
DAC	Development Assistance Committee (OECD)
EID	New, Emerging, and Re-emerging Infectious Diseases
EMC	Division of Emerging and other Communicable Diseases Surveillance and Control (WHO)
GAVI	Global Alliance for Vaccines and Immunization
GOARN	Global Outbreak Alert and Response Network (WHO)
GPHIN	Global Public Health Intelligence Network
IHR	International Health Regulations
IOM	Institute of Medicine (USA)
ISR	International Sanitary Regulations
LCDC	Laboratory Centre for Disease Control (Canada)
NCID	National Center for Infectious Diseases (USA)
NIH	National Institutes of Health (USA)
OECD	Organization for Economic Co-operation and Development
PAHO	Pan American Health Organization
PHAC	Public Health Agency of Canada

PEPFAR   U.S. President's Emergency Plan For AIDS Relief

SARS   Severe Acute Respiratory Syndrome

TB   Tuberculosis

UK   United Kingdom

US(A)   United States (of America)

WHA   World Health Assembly

WHO   World Health Organization

Acknowledgments

Alan Hunt and Alison Bashford shouldered the collegial task of reviewing the proposal for what became this book. We hope that they are pleased with the result as we took their comments to heart.

A number of our colleagues made friendly contributions. The benefits of collegial relations are manifold, a perception that especially comes to mind in the context of research writing rather than department meetings.

Lorna would like to thank Brian Singer for his careful reading and invaluable comments on Chapter 5, wherein she in part takes up the problematic of the relation between governance and sovereignty in articles that he and she have coauthored. Frank Pearce was an interlocutor throughout, commenting on drafts and offering valuable editorial advice. The results of stimulating conversations with Barbara Godard are found at many places in this book, as is her editorial advice. Majella Coleman and Karen Schucher provided immensely helpful listening skills at many junctures. Fuyuki Kurasawa forwarded valuable briefing documents related to his work with Daniel Cefaï on what they have termed contemporary French "pragmatic sociology." An inspirational e-mail exchange with Craig McFarlane on algorithms is partially reflected in our comments here, although further work on algorithmic practices needs doing.

Eric would like to thank Michael Bresalier for his insights about the very possibility for a rigorous historical and social analysis of emerging infectious diseases. He provided invaluable suggestions regarding the scholarly and popular literatures on emerging infectious diseases and was a most valued listener to and commenter on early formulations of this book. With her characteristic enthusiasm and goodwill Joan Eakin provided just the kind of encouragement required for thinking through how to fashion an analysis of global emergency vigilance as a contribution to a sociology of public health. In a series of conversations, Liza McCoy helped to clarify the significance of our research site for studies in the social organization of knowledge. Todd Sherman provided encouragement and support and a thoughtful ear throughout the writing process. Chris Sanders offered his usual professionalism and exactitude in a number of research assistance tasks over the course of the project.

We would both like to thank Alan Boutilier and Barbara Godard who contributed their expertise as translators to our work here. We are grateful for their help and owe them dinner.

Albert Banerjee served as the main research assistant to our work. We will long remember his sharp intelligence, steady support, and exceptional research skills.

We both thank our research participants at WHO (Geneva), GPHIN (Ottawa), and Factiva (Toronto) for taking the time from their busy schedules to speak with us. Abla Mawudeku (GPHIN) was most generous, facilitating our access to GPHIN and providing us with careful, time-consuming readings of our analysis of the GPHIN system. David Heymann (WHO) treated two social scientists with a new interest in global public health with complete respect and paved our way to interviews at WHO without which this book would not have been written.

Librarians at York University (Toronto) and the WHO Library (Geneva) were generous with their time in support of our historical research. We thank Sharona Brookman and Daniel Perlin, reference librarians at Osgoode Hall, Law School of York University, for help with our searches related to the history of international health law. Avril Reid at the WHO Library (Geneva) and Marie Villemin at WHO Records and Archives always had precise and ready answers for our many research questions.

The writing and research for this project were carried out by the two authors as follows: Chapters 1, 2, 5 and 6 were cowritten with Weir as the lead author. Chapter 4 was cowritten with Mykhalovskiy as lead. Chapter 3 was a joint effort. In the early stages of the project, the authors worked together on its analytical, theoretical, and methodological frameworks. The interview and archival research was jointly conducted. In the latter stages of the project Weir took an overall leadership role in writing and in bringing the manuscript to completion.

Mykhalovskiy's involvement in the project was facilitated by a Canadian Institutes of Health Research New Investigator Award (Institute of Infection and Immunity [HIV/AIDS]—Health Services/Population Health Stream). Weir's work on the project was partially supported by a Social Sciences and Humanities Council of Canada Standard Research Grant, "Biosecurity and Synthetic Biology," which she holds. We would like to thank Health Care, Technology, and Place (Canadian Institutes for Health Research Strategic Training Initiative in Health Research) for their funding of this project through an ICE grant that we jointly held. A number of internal funds at York University supported this project: a Faculty of Arts Start-up Grant for new faculty held by Mykhalovskiy and Faculty of Arts, SSHRC Small, and SSHRC Grant in Aid of Travel grants held by Weir. We are grateful to all these agencies and funds for their research support.

Lorna Weir
Eric Mykhalovskiy

1 Knowing Global Public Health

Infectious diseases have again become culturally fascinating to the peoples of the global North. Avian flu and swine flu are endlessly newsworthy topics. Novels and nonfiction books about epidemics become best sellers. Films about fictionalized contagious disease outbreaks attract audiences who have acquired a taste for being scared by really nasty bugs.

The present book is a study in another aspect of this interest in infectious diseases: public health expertise, specifically changes that have occurred since the late 1990s in how international public health authorities come to know about internationally significant infectious disease outbreaks and other emergencies. Whereas prior to the mid-1990s the World Health Organization (WHO) was charged with preventing the international transmission of a small number of infectious diseases,[1] today global public health security targets the much more expansive target of international public health emergencies. We seek to understand this very recent historical break in global public health by analyzing the transformation in international communicable disease control in terms of three processes: (1) the impact of a new disease concept called 'emerging infectious diseases' (EID), (2) the invention of a monitoring/surveillance technique called 'online early warning outbreak detection,' and (3) the formation of a politico-juridical regime dealing with international public health emergencies.

Our interest in contemporary global public health knowledge of infectious disease outbreaks and other health emergencies was sparked by the 2003 SARS outbreak in Toronto, Canada. We each initially knew SARS through TV, radio, talking with friends, and contacts with public health officials. Weir, who lives in Toronto, also experienced the reactions of people local to the outbreak by speaking with family members of those who were ill, noticing hospital measures for infectious disease control, and seeing fewer people in restaurants. We observed that our experiences of SARS in Toronto and in Halifax, Canada (where Mykhalovskiy lived at the time) were mediated through local and global news reports that presented us with images of Canadian public health officials in dialogue with WHO, the latter coordinating global efforts to control SARS. In Canada, the SARS outbreak precipitated debate about the political effects of travel advisories and the evidentiary basis upon which are based public health judgments about issuing and lifting them (Kraus 2003). It also spurred widespread discussion about the processes for identifying and responding to infectious disease outbreaks that, like SARS, can quickly traverse the globe.

This book represents our collaborative effort to understand how infectious disease outbreaks and other events currently come into knowledge within global public health. It is the result of an intellectual and research journey that began with our conversations in Toronto about SARS and continued into our meeting and interviewing officials at WHO in Geneva together with research at the WHO Library and Archives. Along the way we interviewed public health officials at the Global Public Health Intelligence Network (GPHIN) based in Ottawa, Canada, and wrestled with the complex technical innovations that they and others had introduced into contemporary international infectious disease monitoring. We read international and Canadian government reports about the SARS outbreak that emphasized the need to improve how outbreaks and emergencies are identified and acted on both domestically and globally. We attended national and international conferences on infectious diseases in Australia, Canada, Europe, and the USA. We learned about new concepts such as 'emerging infectious diseases' and 'public health emergencies of international concern,' read about global health governance, and waded through the impressive historical and contemporary work on international infectious disease control. We also struggled with the available frameworks for understanding current public health governance arrangements as we sought to make sense of our research object.

Throughout the process, we were struck by the paucity of sociological attention to contemporary international infectious disease control, particularly when compared to the corpus of work produced by historians and those working from political science and international law perspectives. Public health is not an uncommon focus of sociological research, but sociological work addressing public health practices at the global level and particularly at the level of international infectious disease control remains a rarity. We were also surprised by how new practices in international infectious disease control and emergency governance played out against a background of shifting public health concepts and ways of knowing that had not been fully identified or explored by existing research. We wrote this book to respond to these absences and intend it to be a sociological contribution to research on contemporary global public health with an emphasis on the analysis of knowledge relations.

In thinking and writing about knowledge in the context of global public health, our collaboration has created a dialogue between two traditions of inquiry sensitive to the analysis of discourse, concepts, and the formal apparatus of expertise and knowledge: the history of the present (from the work of Michel Foucault) and studies in the social organization of knowledge (from the work of Canadian sociologist Dorothy Smith). While we discuss that dialogue more fully in the following section, we have found that working across these two traditions has made us sensitive to the productivity of knowledge at a social and institutional level. Our analytic stance takes up knowledge as a constituent of the social that shapes how things are done, including how they get done at the level of large-scale relations such as those of global public health. In this book we explore how conceptual shifts and new uses of knowledge have driven change and created new possibilities for action within the technical and political arrangements of what we have come to call 'global public health emergency vigilance.'

We use the phrase global public health emergency vigilance, or more usually the shorter and less cumbersome 'global emergency vigilance' or 'emergency vigilance' to conceptualize the object of our study, doing so with an approach that is oriented primarily to the study of knowledge. The goal of global public health emergency vigilance is to recognize dangers to public health, verify information, send alerts, and intervene before a situation becomes internationally catastrophic. In the world on alert for international public health emergencies, the watchful apparatus of emergency vigilance detects the marginal and dangerous event.

Emergency vigilance marks a deep revision in public health reasoning, a reconstruction and displacement of infectious disease control. Global emergency vigilance differs from the previous period of international infectious disease control in its target (main antagonist), goal, relation to the potential, conceptualization of report, temporal modality, and securitization.

International health law in the 20th century targeted infectious diseases, whereas current international health law in force since 2007 targets "international public health emergencies." International public health emergency includes but is not confined to infectious diseases, instead extending to anything that crosses international boundaries and damages human health at a population level. The public health aspects of chemical, industrial, environmental, and radiological disasters may be international emergencies as indeed may be infectious disease outbreaks of yellow fever or Marburg hemorrhagic fever.

The goal of global emergency vigilance is to contain public health emergencies prior to their spread across international boundaries rather than, as previously, to interrupt the international transmission of infectious diseases after they had crossed an international boundary. Global emergency vigilance aims to detect the wide range of emerging and potential diseases and medical conditions rather than, as was the case throughout the 20th century, actual cases of known diseases. The period of emergency vigilance orients to both the potential and the actual.

The transition to emergency vigilance also transformed the conceptualization of report, both what was to be reported to WHO and who was qualified to do such reporting. Whereas the prior period of international infectious disease control required that national public health officials report to WHO *cases* of infectious diseases, emergency vigilance requires the reporting of *events*. Case reports were of disease diagnoses. "Event" is a broader concept that refers to the appearance of a disease or something that "creates the potential for disease;" the concept of "disease" is extended to include both illnesses and medical conditions such as injury (International Health Regulations [IHR] 2005: Definitions). Events are reported not only by sovereign states, but also by online outbreak detection systems and nonstate organizations that draw on unofficial sources of information, such as global health news.

With respect to temporal modality, global emergency vigilance holds itself to a standard of operating in 'real time;' public health knowledge is to coincide with the time in which the emergency is occurring to facilitate flexible public health actions. During the previous period, WHO's knowledge of epidemics did not synchronize with their occurrence. Many epidemics were simply local events unknown to national and international authorities. WHO was often not notified of outbreaks that required report under international law because of the economic consequences of doing so for the country involved. The result was that WHO only became aware of some epidemics long after the initial outbreak.

Lastly, the juridical relations of international public health emergencies have, unlike all previous forms of international health law that applied only to a small number of known infectious diseases, been extended to apply to the public health aspects of accidental and deliberate chemical, biological, radiological and nuclear incidents. Emergency vigilance has thus been securitized in the sense of articulating global public health with international security—the relations across sovereign states together with treaties and institutions that structure the transstate relations.

Global emergency vigilance is implicated in one of the great political questions of our present: the constitution of a political level beyond national sovereignty. The requirement that emergency vigilance have the earliest possible knowledge of actual, emerging, and potential events challenged the postcolonial flows of public health knowledge, specifically that the ultimate place of power over international infectious disease reporting to WHO was a sovereign matter, and sovereigns could refuse to report with impunity. In the name of a potential/virtual microbial world and heightened detection standards, a new world order in health was fashioned at the turn of the 21st century that emancipated public health knowledge from its subordination to sovereignty and constituted WHO as a power above the sovereign. We argue that global emergency vigilance illustrates the insufficiency of any theory that would reduce the political to either sovereignty or to governance. It is precisely the form of the political beyond both governance and sovereignty that is raised at the site of global emergency vigilance.

Our writing here is intended as a contribution to the understanding of global biopolitics. The concept of biopolitics refers to an historical change—an epochal one—that began in the 18th century and continues to date. In Foucault's words, "biopolitics"/"biopower" was a "general strategy of power" whereby "starting from the eighteenth century, modern societies took on board the fundamental biological fact that human beings are a species" (Foucault 2007: 1). Global emergency vigilance is biopolitical in this sense because it aims at the conservation of populations and citizens within and across sovereign states. It has a double and inconsistent logic, one of containing emergencies from spreading into the North, but also a cosmopolitan one of securing human health for all the peoples of the world.

This is a theoretico-empirical book in which theory, analysis, and the empirical mutually enable and limit one another, although it begins in the empirical and ends in the theoretical. The central analytic intent of our research is to explore the significance of changes in knowledge for the emergence of a new global public health apparatus. Our topic, global public health emergency vigilance, involves an international apparatus that links human actors, technologies, microbial phenomena, political powers, laws, forms of knowledge, and organizations. We have taken care to give proper due to the complex technical developments and shifts in knowledge represented by global emergency vigilance, but we do so in ways that contribute to our central analytic interest in knowledge as active.

At many times during the writing of this book we were forcefully struck by the commitment among those with whom we spoke to public health for those in the global South and the global North. We deeply respect their work. At the same time, we are keenly conscious of the limitations of and problems inherent in current global public health security, which clearly has been primarily driven by the North. To say this is not to discount the stated positions of public health officials from Asia and Africa who have told us unequivocally that emerging infectious diseases and international public health emergencies are concerns of the South as well as the North. We, however, follow the historian and philosopher Foucault in being more interested in the explication of the dangerous than in judgments of the good and bad.

Global Public Health Emergency Vigilance

We came to the concept of global emergency vigilance after a long process of considering possibilities for a reflexive naming of our object, a process marked by an awareness of how a name shapes what can be thought about a phenomenon and a concern to find a way of writing that would reflect the analytic specificity of the approach we took to our topic. Few alternatives presented themselves to us. In the health sciences literature, for example, commentators are fond of announcing a new era in global infectious disease control but offer no way of analytically specifying that era. They simply distinguish the new from the old by drawing attention to the greater speed of the current system of global infectious disease control or by identifying other characteristics, such as its challenge to state control over information or its uses of unofficial information, that are then taken as self-evidently new without historical comparison. By turns we considered framing our research object as surveillance and post-Westphalian governance before coming to consider it as a vigilance apparatus.

A) Surveillance?

It would have been more conventional to conceptualize our research as investigating surveillance rather than vigilance. However, our focus is not on detection but on the broader field of relations linking the idea of emerging infectious diseases (EID), the technique of outbreak detection, and the invention of a new politico-juridical framework for global public health emergencies. We wish to examine the field of relations across EID, outbreak detection, and international law rather than frame our discussion in terms of outbreak detection as a surveillance form. Second, if we had chosen surveillance as an explanatory category, it would have been conflated with the public health sense of surveillance. We are well aware that social scientific language cannot be fully separated from the language(s) of its research participants; social scientific studies always bear the accent of their research sites. Yet the use of surveillance saturates the speech practices of our empirical site, making it very difficult to separate sociological from public health senses of surveillance. This would have resulted in conceptual incoherence. In this book, 'surveillance' will be used in its contemporary public health sense to mean collecting, interpreting, disseminating, and acting on health information by authorities.[2]

We have also been reluctant to use surveillance as an explanatory category for analytic reasons. Surveillance studies focus on the human subject. Thus, by way of example, the sociologist David Lyon defines surveillance as " . . . paying very close attention to personal details—often in the form of digital data—for the purpose of influencing, managing, or controlling those under scrutiny" (Lyon 2003: 15). A great deal of the sociology of surveillance has explored the routine, automated gathering of personal data for marketing and security (private and public; local, national, and international). However, online early warning detection does not track personal data. Nor is it restricted to persons. Early warning outbreak detection orients to what is called the "event" in the WHO International Health Regulations (IHR): "a manifestation of disease or an occurrence that creates a potential for a disease" (IHR 2005: Art. 1). Detection of events extends to species other than the human, to environmental disasters, to nuclear explosions, and to the deliberate spread of pathogens. Event detection does not risk-profile individuals, and if anything it lightens the significance of national borders in order to enhance the international public health control of infectious disease outbreaks. Thus the concept of surveillance provided little help in conceptualizing our object of study.

B) Post-Westphalian Governance?

We secondly considered identifying our research object in the politico-juridical terms suggested by David Fidler. Fidler has reflexively named current arrangements in international infectious disease control as a post-Westphalian system of infectious disease governance. A professor of law at Indiana University, Fidler writes on international disease control from the perspective of international legal policy. His work is prodigious, important, and largely defines the field. Fidler (2004b: 42–68) describes international infectious disease control practices associated with the SARS outbreak as post-Westphalian because of the challenge they pose to the previous political system for international disease control that rested fundamentally on state sovereignty. Westphalia in this context refers to the Peace of Westphalia (1648) that ended the Thirty Years War in Europe (a period of religious strife among Christian sects) by establishing a system of equal sovereigns that exercise absolute power within their territories. The Peace of Westphalia brought a formal end to the Holy Roman Empire when formerly feudal powers were no longer required to owe allegiance to the Pope. Westphalia is acknowledged as the moment of crystallization for the principle of state sovereignty within Europe, constituting an international system of sovereign states and their nonsovereign colonial possessions.

Fidler's concept of post-Westphalian public health governance analytically privileges the question of state sovereignty. This is an entirely reasonable thing to do, especially for someone writing from an international law and international relations perspective. Challenges to sovereign state control over knowledge of outbreaks and other public health emergencies have been clearly prominent features of global public health since the mid-1990s. But from our perspective as historically informed social scientists, to characterize the late 20th century transformation of international infectious disease control as post-Westphalian is partial in a number of ways. Fidler has not examined the relation between the Westphalian system and the history of colonialism (Anghie 2007). He treats the Westphalian system of infectious disease control as originating in Italian city-states during the 14th century, continuing through the international sanitary conferences in the second half of the 19th century, effectively ending only at the end of the 20th century (Fidler 2004b: 26–32). This is a fundamentally Eurocentric view that does not ask about the place of colonial public health practices in the Westphalian system of international disease control. As historians such as Lenore Manderson (1995) have shown, information about infectious disease epidemics was under colonial control prior to the formation of the World Health Organization in 1946. Sovereign control over infectious disease information came into practice for Euro-American colonies in the period of decolonization that followed World War II. The Westphalian moment in international disease control thus has a dual periodization, one for the colonizers and one for the colonized. However, we agree with Fidler that the period of Westphalian governance in international infectious disease control came to a de facto end for all WHO country members in the final years of the 20th century, though not legally so until 2004/2005.

We seek to extend Fidler's (2004b: 60–68) account of the relations between official and unofficial information about outbreak during what he terms the Westphalian and post-Westphalian periods. As a specialist in international law and policy, Fidler's historical account of the West-phalian period centers on the history of treaties and formal organizations. Although Fidler (2001: 845) does acknowledge the presence of nongovern-mental actors such as the Rockefeller Foundation and the International Union Against Tuberculosis in international public health between 1851 and 1951, his treatment of unofficial epidemiological communications prior to 1995 is limited to WHO's 1970 announcement of a cholera outbreak in Guinea without official authorization by the Guinean state (Fidler 2004b: 64–65). In an account limited to formal law, it is difficult to see the social relations about which law is silent. As social scientists we are trained to be sensitive to these vast domains of legal silence. Thus, it was important to us as sociologists to investigate the place of news in unofficial epidemiological communications prior to the invention of outbreak detection and to com-pare the differing relations between official and unofficial epidemiological communications before and after the invention of global emergency vigi-lance. Unofficial communications did not spring into existence during the late 1990s. We thus find the concepts of Westphalian and post-Westphalian international public health governance insightful but not ultimately satisfy-ing given our social scientific interest in theorizing the power/knowledge relations of contemporary international public health emergencies.

C) Vigilance

Rather than framing contemporary global infectious disease control as surveillance or as primarily post-Westphalian, we prefer to concep-tualize it as a vigilance apparatus. Vigilance directs analytic attention to apparatuses that continuously monitor phenomena that may give rise to catastrophic events. In the public health sense, vigilance refers to an attitude of being attentive, alert, and watchful; vigilance is an ethical standard to be used by public health officials in the course of their work. The meaning of vigilance we use here is a sociological one introduced by Chateauraynaud and Torny (1999) in *Les sombres précurseurs: Une sociologie pragmatique de l'alerte et du risque*. They argue that vigilance apparatuses were a state response in the second half of the 20th century to political pressures to take care of health, the environment, and lifestyle in the face of ongoing dangers from diverse sources such as nuclear energy and contamination of groundwater (Chateauraynaud & Torny 1999: 29). Since the 1960s a number of vigilance apparatuses have been established to monitor events thought to be precursors of catastrophic incidents. Vigilance is a watchful apparatus that produces a stream of monitoring data in order to identify singular cases; the cases are subject to verification, and if verified, alerts are issued. Vigilance and alert systems are a form of social action oriented to foresight (Chateauraynaud & Torny 1999: 415). The concept of vigilance is in part situated in a long trajectory of scholarship that has explored state and governmental action for the protection and conservation of popular health (Bock & Thane 1991; Foucault 1979/1997; Skocpol 1992).

The vigilance apparatus concept formulated by Chateauraynaud and Torny is located in a sociological research trajectory that has been concerned with analyzing the ways in which advanced modernity envisions the future in order to act on it in the present. The many social science studies of risk systems are part of this research trajectory, as are recent studies of the precautionary principle in contemporary policy (Ewald 2002) and governing through uncertainty (O'Malley 2004; Power 2007). Chateauraynaud and Torny (1999: 77–78) counterpose vigilance apparatuses to the precautionary principle. The precautionary principle is invoked to prohibit activities that are regarded as potentially catastrophic (e.g., the dangers of nuclear power indicate the need to abolish the nuclear power industry). In contrast to the precautionary principle, vigilance apparatuses permit the continued operation of dangerous industries through a fine-grained system of monitoring and alerts. Vigilance begins when precaution has been politically foreclosed. Thus, vigilance apparatuses form a technical means that the political economies of high modernity have found to coexist with the dangers they have created—dangers that include the cases of asbestos, bovine spongiform encephalopathy (BSE), and nuclear power discussed by Chateauraynaud and Torny.

We differ from Chateauraynaud and Torny in arguing for a distinction between vigilance apparatuses and risk techniques. Unlike risk techniques, vigilance apparatuses are not intrinsically calculative—though they sometimes are—as they aim to identify the specific, suspicious event that is distinguished from a background of prior data. Vigilance apparatuses operate through exhaustive sensitivity, whereas risk systems act by estimating the likelihood of unwanted future harms based on the calculation of probabilities (Ewald 1991: 202; Weir 2006: 16–19). For instance, automobile insurance is a risk system: The cost of individual auto insurance is based on estimates of the number of accidents that will occur over a year; the expenses associated with the resulting claims are then distributed over the risk pool of insured persons. Vigilance is about detection, alert, and response rather than predictive calculation of probabilities. It is directed at detecting harm rather than estimating the risk of harm. Risk and vigilance are separate techniques of foresight.

Chateauraynaud and Torny undertake what they term a "pragmatic sociology of alert and risk." Their book is aligned with a general movement in contemporary French sociology away from structuralism and Bourdieu's critical sociology and toward many of the concerns that characterized the North American recovery from structural functionalism: social interaction, context, meaning making, and experience (Cefaï 2008; Cefaï & Kurasawa 2008).[3] The best known of this intellectual work within the Anglophone world has been the actor–network theory of Michel Callon and Bruno Latour in the sociology of science, but pragmatic sociology extends far beyond actor–network theory. Pragmatic sociology has engaged with the social interactionism of Goffman and the ethnomethodology of Garfinkel as well as U.S. philosophical pragmatism, particularly the figures of William James, John Dewey, and George Herbert Mead. Dewey's *The Public and Its Problems* has been influential in framing a trajectory of inquiry about the formation of civic groups and the constitution of public problems. Chateauraynaud and Torny's *Les sombres précurseurs* reflects the interest of pragmatic sociology in situated action and the contested space of public problems.

But the lineage of our work lies elsewhere than pragmatic sociology in the history of the present and studies in the social organization of knowledge (outlined in the following section of this chapter) and their common concern for knowledge and its relation to power. So too, where Chateauraynaud and Torny's emphasis falls on risk and alerts as social action and public contestations around their legitimacy, our work has foregrounded the formation of an international vigilance apparatus that integrates issuing alerts as one of its many functions. Chateauraynaud and Torny's conception of vigilance as a watchful apparatus that stands on guard and manages crises (1999: 15) is the aspect of their work that has been the most useful to our own. For our purposes, vigilance is in part helpful because it breaks from the assumption that the social is immediately known by those who enact it. Vigilance is a sociological concept that departs from the understandings expertise has of its own practices.

Following the conventions of pragmatic sociology, we understand emergency vigilance to be an apparatus in a sociological sense: a network of heterogeneous elements linking human actors, objects, statements, and technical devices. But the vigilance apparatus investigated here is an international one, unlike the national apparatuses examined by Chateauraynaud and Torny. Global emergency vigilance implicated political and legal questions of world order. Bringing global emergency vigilance into the sphere of juridical right required major revisions to international public health law. Global emergency vigilance posed political questions of how WHO was authorized to know about public health emergencies and where the ultimate place of power in international public health lay, whether with sovereign states or with WHO.

The global emergency vigilance apparatus is comprised of four main social actions: outbreak detection, verification, alert, and response. Its institutional network is led by Epidemic and Pandemic Alert and Response at WHO headquarters that coordinates WHO Regional Offices, the national focal points mandated under the IHR (2005) to act as communication contacts, and the international network of WHO partners in the Global Outbreak Alert and Response Network (GOARN). The establishment of this institutional network was initially led by the Division of Emerging and Other Communicable Diseases Surveillance and Response at WHO headquarters, a unit that was established in October 1995. During the period between 1998 and 2003, the formation of the vigilance apparatus was centered in the work of the Division of Communicable Diseases Cluster at WHO (headed by David Heymann), particularly its Communicable Disease Surveillance and Response (CSR) unit.

What we have conceptualized as a global vigilance apparatus was and is inserted in a broader WHO programme of communicable disease prevention, control, and eradication practices. These include efforts to control HIV/AIDS, TB, malaria, neglected tropical diseases, and vaccine research and development. The emergency vigilance apparatus was made part of broader communicable disease efforts by WHO in the context of renewed emphasis on communicable disease control that began in the second half of the 1990s.

D) Outbreak or Emergency?

While drafting this book, we initially conceptualized what we were studying as global 'outbreak' vigilance rather than 'emergency' vigilance. 'Outbreak' is much used in contemporary public health as a synonym for 'epidemic,' each conceptualized as a higher-than-usual incidence of a disease in a population. Last's *Dictionary of Epidemiology* (Last 2001), a standard reference work sponsored by the International Epidemiological Association, identifies outbreak as a local epidemic. The Centers for Disease Control and Prevention (CDC) uses 'outbreak' and 'epidemic' synonymously, though it recommends 'outbreak' be used in dealings with the public for purposes of reassurance (Dato, Shephard, & Wagner 2006: 24). But there are in practice qualitative distinctions in the usages of outbreak and epidemic, with outbreaks considered a "window of opportunity" prior to epidemic, though difficult to spot because they are "silent" and may "sicken or kill individuals before they are detected" (Wagner 2006: 1). The concept of outbreak is used to fashion an interval prior to epidemic when it can be contained. The concept of outbreak may be applied to both infectious and noninfectious diseases; there can, for instance, be an outbreak of liver cancer although it is not considered infectious. 'Outbreak vigilance' thus seemed to be the very concept we needed.

Ultimately we realized that outbreak vigilance would not suffice because outbreak applies only to diseases, communicable and noncommunicable. The research terrain we were investigating targeted more than diseases. For instance, online detection tracks international environmental and industrial disasters wherein people are injured or poisoned. The main target of the IHR (2005) is not infectious disease as was the case with all previous international health law, but rather "public health emergencies of international concern," a concept that is not disease specific. As we began to understand the depth of the epistemological and organizational shift in public health that we were investigating, 'emergency vigilance' seemed to us more accurate than 'outbreak vigilance' because the term emergency applies to both diseases and conditions. Emergency vigilance better expresses the move to a problem-space that includes but is not restricted to infectious diseases.

After the passage of the IHR (2005) it made little sense to call public health activities dealing with international public health emergencies by the older term 'communicable disease control,' and terminology at WHO began to reference 'public health security' and 'human security.' In the 2007 World Health Report, *A Safer Future: Global Public Health Security in the 21st Century*, Director-General of WHO Margaret Chan glosses global public health security as "the reduced vulnerability of populations to acute threats to health" (WHO 2007: 3). Security implicates far more than disease outbreaks. Emergency vigilance, we argue, is linked with two meanings of security. One sense, human security, involves sustaining and promoting the conditions for human life and, in the words of the WHO Constitution, human well-being. In another sense of security, emergency vigilance has been integrated into international security, seeking to protect the international order against the public health aspects of infectious diseases and a wide range of emergencies caused by the use of chemical, biological, radiological, and nuclear weapons.

E) These Chapters

In Chapter 2 we explore how the invention and internationalization of the EID concept—new, emerging, and re-emerging infectious diseases—produced an epistemological shift in public health that provided the initial impetus to the formation of global emergency vigilance. The EID concept was fashioned in the U.S. context during the years 1989 through 1992 as a challenge to diminished interest in and funding for infectious disease control. The EID concept was explicitly linked to U.S. national security concerns and constructed infectious disease as a "microbial threat" to the USA that would require a renewal of the public health system after decades of neglect.

From the first, the EID concept was applied not only to known diseases, but also to unknown, unnamed, and potential infectious diseases. Over the course of its internationalization and recontextualization from the USA to WHO headquarters in the mid-1990s, the EID concept established a pervasive presence in international public health circles. The EID concept caught the imagination of public health officials as it coordinated in a single concept the possibility of constant microbial genetic change, the intentional spread of pathogens, ecological spreading, and a frightening future of unknown diseases. It so successfully harnessed public health anxieties (particularly in the global North) about transnationally mobile microbes that it came to discursively structure a call for spectacular changes in the speed and reach of global communicable disease identification and response. The EID concept remade international communicable disease control, operating as the discursive target for a new way of knowing and acting on communicable disease outbreaks that appears in the WHO vision of a "world on alert" (WHO 1996), the constitutive metaphor for global emergency vigilance.

In Chapter 3 we explore how the demand for earlier and more comprehensive EID detection problematized existing public health surveillance during the mid-1990s. Our analysis of online early warning outbreak detection focuses on changes in the organizational presence of news reports in the processes through which outbreaks and related public health events are detected and verified. We compare the place of news in epidemiological communications about outbreak before and after the invention of online early warning outbreak detection. We show that news, an unofficial knowledge of outbreak, had long been part of international epidemiological communications prior to the 1990s. WHO personnel also had official knowledge of outbreak communicated through the reports of its country members. Unofficial information such as news was often faster than official country reports and contained information about outbreaks that sovereign states did not report.

In order to meet the demand for faster knowledge of outbreak and what later, in the first years of the 21st century, came to be defined as international public health emergencies, public health officials interiorized online health news as an information source within the global apparatus of infectious disease control. They invented a new technique for identification of and response to outbreak, called online early warning outbreak detection and alert, that principally drew on news for the identification of outbreaks and public health events. Although news had been incorporated in public health knowledge of outbreak decades prior to the 1990s, the invention of early warning outbreak detection changed the methods for identifying, collecting, analyzing, and acting on news reports. Under conditions of early warning outbreak detection and alert, what public health officials had previously drawn upon only sporadically became, in its electronic and 'near real-time' form, a standardized information resource. Early warning outbreak detection was an historic development in the knowledge relations of international infectious disease control. It had dramatic consequences for the international legal framework that governed global communication of information about outbreak.

Every vigilance apparatus exists in a political and regulatory context that authorizes its existence and actions. In the case of emergency vigilance this context is international, unlike the national (France and UK) case studies that are the focus of Chateauraynaud and Torny's book. In Chapter 4 we explore the politico-juridical framework that was precipitated by the EID concept and the use of early warning outbreak detection and alert. We draw particular attention to the new legal concepts of 'public health event' and 'public health emergency' introduced in the IHR (2005) that broke with a long history of limiting the object of legally mandated notification to lists of infectious diseases. Political pressures on WHO to deal with EID propelled the formulation of legal concepts that would define mandatory reporting requirements in such a way as to encompass the unknown, the uncertain, and the potential, rather than only actual, named diseases. The conceptual shifts made in the IHR (2005) meant that public health systems that had been familiar with the concept of reporting cases or suspected cases of a disease were now required to report on events, a new and expansive category. We explore how the IHR (2005) seek to stabilize the translocal meaning of event through the inclusion within the Regulations of two new interpretive devices: an algorithm (a decision tree) for identifying events that may constitute international public health emergencies and an accompanying guide (IHR 2005: Annex 2). We argue that the IHR (2005) dispensed with the disease list as a statement form, introducing the algorithm and guide to provide a grid of intelligibility for international public health emergencies.

The relation of global emergency vigilance to the political is taken up in Chapter 5. In the name of the dangers posed by global public health emergencies, a reconstitution of the political in global biopolitics took place. WHO acquired powers beyond those of its sovereign Member States when the governance apparatus for emergency vigilance, an apparatus formed extralegally in the period between 1998 and 2003, was given legal mandate in the IHR (2005). International health law emancipated outbreak knowledge from sovereign power, enabled the knowledge relations necessary for the governance of the potential and the actual, and formed for the first time a suprasovereign political power in global biopolitics.

Rather than analyze global biopolitics as having only one level—the governmental—we suggest that it be theorized as having three aspects: governance, sovereignty, and a suprasovereign level of power organized around a symbolic conception of a common fate in public health. This conception of biopolitics rejects the reduction of the political to governance on the grounds that it leaves no way of understanding some of what is most dangerous in our present, including the proliferation of governance without political accountability outside the sphere of juridical right. The constitution of the political beyond governance is one of the great political stakes and tasks of our time. Social and political theory has an ethical work of the first importance in conceptualizing the political beyond global governance, much as did the political theorists of the early modern period in theorizing state sovereignty and public law.

Revitalizing the Sociology of Public Health

This book seeks to substantively and conceptually revitalize the sociology of public health. Substantively we examine recent transformations in international infectious disease control, a topic that has received no sociological commentary to date. Conceptually we seek to understand the significance of knowledge, particularly new public health concepts and techniques, in the constitution of a global emergency vigilance apparatus at the turn of the 21st century. We use a sociology of knowledge, one that is sensitive to social organization, as the basis of our analysis. The sociology of knowledge we use is one formed in a dialogue between the history of the present (Foucauldian research) and studies in the social organization of knowledge. This analytic approach distinguishes our work from most social scientists in the field of global health who tend to focus on social inequalities in the distribution of health and illness (Kickbusch 2006; Navarro 2007). Another stream of social science research seeks to establish health as a human right and a global public good (Chen, Evans, & Cash 1999; R. Smith, Beaglehole, & Woodward 2003). While we are sympathetic to the normative orientation of such work, our own research problematic is knowledge and knowledge relations in global emergency vigilance.

Substantively we have been struck by the limited social science engagement with contemporary infectious disease control and, more broadly, global public health. Those social scientists who have written about global public health and international infectious disease control have primarily been political scientists in the fields of international relations (Zacher & Keefe 2008; Kaul, Grunberg, & Stern 1999) and in the just developing field of global health governance (Aginam 2005b; Kickbusch 2000, 2002, 2003a, 2003b; Lee 2003; Lee, Buse, & Fustukian 2002; Zacher & Keefe 2008). Given our own backgrounds in fields that are sensitive to knowledge relations—Weir in the history of the present and Mykhalovskiy in studies in the social organization of knowledge—our work in the present book tries to open global emergency vigilance to sociological consideration with a particular emphasis on the social analysis of knowledge.

A) The Sociology of Public Health: An Overview

It is common to understand sociology's relationship to public health as structured around a central tension between research in the service of public health and research that criticizes its assumptions, policies, and practices. Yet the distinction between sociology *in* public health versus *of* public health surely obscures the complexity and range of sociological engagement with public health. Sociologists have produced a breadth of work on various questions related to public health drawing on multiple theoretical and methodological perspectives and often commingling applied and critical pursuits. Recent sociological interventions in public health research on social inequalities foregrounding concepts such as social capital (Turner 2003; Coburn 2000; Wakefield & Poland 2005) and collective lifestyles (Frohlich, Corin, & Potvin 2001) and sociological commentary on global public health interventions such as male circumcision for HIV/AIDS prevention (Dowsett & Couch 2007) and strategies for addressing "obesity" (Campos 2004; Mitchell & McTigue 2007) belie simple classification as either *in* or *of* public health.

While the distinction between sociology *in* versus *of* public health can be overwrought, in a more nuanced form it can help suggest contours of important differences in how sociological research orients to established public health reasoning and practice. At a time when state research funding in multiple national contexts aggressively promotes applied health research (Mykhalovskiy et al. 2008; Learmonth 2003), the in/of distinction can help point to the challenges of formulating and maintaining a space for independent intellectual inquiry about public health; it should not be fully discarded.

Our research on global emergency vigilance is fashioned as a commentary on recent developments in its knowledge and knowledge relations. We are not principally concerned to directly contribute to infectious disease control and health security. At the same time, it is not our intent to launch a normative critique of global emergency vigilance. While our work is most broadly located within traditions of sociology that treat public health as an object of inquiry, it is distinguished from the two major research trajectories that define that investigative stance: political economy and Foucauldian studies. In the case of the latter, our work is intended as a renewal and reorientation as Weir herself works from this tradition of inquiry.

Political economy research formulates a strong critique of public health that directs analytic attention to relationships among capital, the state, public health, and civil society; it harkens back to social justice traditions associated with early public health movements. A central argument is that contemporary public health practice accommodates the dominant interests of advanced capitalist societies. A great deal of political economy work on public health is empirically focused on health promotion that is criticized for retreating into a narrow focus on individual, lifestyle health risks rather than taking up an activist direction that would challenge key social, political, and economic institutions (Spitler 2001; Levinson 1998). The emphasis on individual risk factors is further faulted for laying the blame for poor health on individuals, while bypassing the role played by the unequal distribution of economic, social, cultural, and other resources at a societal level (Raphael 2004). In a characteristic liberatory gesture, political economists typically call for a transformed public health, the efforts of which would be directed at mobilizing civil society organizations to lobby the state and otherwise work towards improving housing, education, employment opportunities, and other structural factors affecting the health of communities (Coburn et al. 2003).

A powerful example of political economy's critical engagement with public health can be found in the work on population health discourse by members of the Critical Social Sciences Group based at the University of Toronto. In a series of writings they launched a strong critique of the displacement of health promotion by population health as a leading discourse for thinking about the relationship between health and social determinants in Canada and internationally (Eakin, Robertson, Poland, Coburn, & Edwards 1996; Robertson 1998; Poland et al. 1998; Coburn et al. 2003). Their work, in which Mykhalovskiy has participated, displays a characteristic preoccupation of critical sociologies with recuperating and reclaiming the terrain of 'the social' from its diminished positioning within authoritative public health discourse. Thus, while population health is praised for directing attention to nonmedical influences on general health, it is criticized for ignoring the structural context of health inequalities and reducing questions of social dynamics to the interplay of epidemiologically conceived variables and factors.

Sociological work on 20th century public health informed by Foucauldian analytics is indebted to David Armstrong's important work on historical shifts in medical knowledge in Britain and his analysis of the emergence of new forms of identity associated with the rise of "surveillance medicine" (Armstrong 1983, 1995). Armstrong argued that surveillance medicine remapped the space of illness, turning away from a clinical gaze focused on individual pathological anatomy to the site of "extracorporal" social spaces. Rather than penetrating the interior of human bodies, the new medicine reread symptoms and signs as risk factors for the surveillance of normal populations. Armstrong drew particular attention to the emergence of "lifestyle" and "pre-illness" as sites of public health monitoring (1995: 401).

Armstrong's early insights about new forms of health- and risk-related identity associated with emerging forms of public health was extended in the mid-1990s in work published by the Australian sociologists Alan Petersen and Deborah Lupton (Lupton 1995; Petersen & Lupton 1996) and in contributions to the edited collection *Foucault, Health and Medicine* (Petersen & Bunton 1997). The Australian work characteristically applied a Foucauldian analysis of governance to public health, understanding governance as the "conduct of conduct," that is, the reasoning and techniques developed by state and nonstate expertise to manage human conduct (Miller & Rose 1990: 8). Rather than critiquing public health for failing to adequately address the structural determinants of health like their political economy counterparts, the work of the Australian group drew attention to how public health expertise functioned as a form of moral regulation that constructed and reproduced new experiences of selves and bodies. In particular, these sociologies of public health theorized health promotion as a form of neoliberal governance that sought to manage the subjects of public health by positioning them as interested and responsible for their own health and engaged in the management of their risk factors. Thus was born the active subject in public health.

Our work departs from the foundational principles of political economy and from current work on neoliberal governance by historians of the present. We are sympathetic to critiques of the displacement of public health resources occasioned by EID and by international infectious disease control's relative neglect of the social and economic circumstances that promote infectious disease outbreaks in the first instance. We refuse, however, to reduce the specificity of the object of our study by relegating it to treatment as yet another instance in a long line of public health failures to address social structure. Global emergency vigilance is also ill-suited to the standard Foucauldian analyses of neoliberal governance in public health. Nowhere in our account do we discuss emergency vigilance as a form of governance that interpellates the subject as responsible and active in her/his health practices. Global emergency vigilance does not operate through the active subject. The political and governmental relations of emergency vigilance need a separate analysis from Foucauldian-inspired social science work that explored the 'new public health' and its techniques of health promotion.

Conceptually our work bridges the history of the present and a sociological approach to researching advanced modernity known as studies in the social organization of knowledge first formulated by Dorothy Smith. The possibility of articulating these (in many ways) divergent schools arises from their common interest in examining relations between power and knowledge. Each prizes close analyses of know-how, with the history of the present focusing on discursive apparatuses and studies in the social organization of knowledge on the social practices of ruling. We argue that the history of the present was formulated by Foucault as analytically distinct from the theorization of institutions, social relations, and social processes. From a social scientific perspective, the history of the present is systemically incomplete as it does not provide an account of the realization of discourse at the level of social relations, common culture, or institutional forms.

B) The History of the Present

The history of the present rigorously constructed what to social scientists must appear as a partial object. The main object of the history of the present was formulated by Foucault as the study of learned discourses that are normed by truth (Foucault 1994d: 843–844). Learned discourses comprise "serious" statements that are rare and repeatable, an " . . . ensemble of more or less regulated, more or less conscious, more or less finalized ways of doing things . . ." (Foucault 1998: 463). The claims to truth of these discourses both presuppose and enable plays for power.

In a 1978 exchange with a group of eminent French historians after the publication of his book on the history of French penal practices, *Discipline and Punish* (1979), Foucault clarified his aims and approach to the writing of history. The historian, according to Foucault, studies the prison, delinquency, or French society in a given period, whereas he himself frames inquiry in terms of the history of rational practices (Foucault 1980/1994b: 14–15). More generally, his project is to understand what significance rational practices based on the division true/false have had within Western history (Foucault 1980/1994c: 29–30). Foucault's works investigated *savoirs*—expert knowledges such as criminology and psychology—and scientific *connaissances* such as biology or physics (Weir 2008). Foucault emphasized that he did not seek to investigate the "real in prisons," while maintaining that rational practices have "effects in the real" at the level of institutional practice, individual behavior, and perception (Foucault 1980/1994c: 28–29). The relation between *savoirs* and social institutions is, he argued, one of simplification and uneven distribution, found at some institutional sites but not others. What Foucault called the "rational schemas" of the prison or hospital are "explicit programmes . . . to organize institutions, to design spaces and regulate behaviour" (Foucault 1980/1994c: 27–28). These programmes have effects, but they don't result in societies that completely conform to them (Foucault 1980/1994b: 15–6).

The gap between the "rational schemas" (Foucault 1980/1994c: 27–28) and their realization in the prison or the hospital is an aporia in Foucault's thought—a seemingly obscure point where his thinking becomes incoherent, threatening to undermine his reasoning. This aporia extends to the relations between discipline and a disciplined society, security and a securitized society. We leave this realization problem to the philosophers. From a social scientific perspective it means that Foucault's work will always remain essentially incomplete because social scientists are interested in the realization of rational schemas in institutions, social relations, and social processes, together with the interaction of truthful and nontruthful knowledge.

Because historians of the present sometimes wish to provide an account of how rational schemas and truthful expertise enter into social practice and are realized in speech, some have grafted sociologies, notably actor–network theory, onto Foucauldian analytics (Dean 1996; Miller & Rose 1990; Ong & Collier 2005). Historians of the present have borrowed concepts from actor–network theory as a means of bridging the Foucauldian gap between rational schemas and their realization. Nikolas Rose has suggested "modelling" and "translation" in order to provide a means of thinking about how the alignment between government and conduct is accomplished. Rose uses modelling in two senses: first as the invention of new conceptions of space, and second as "the ways in which acts of government re-implant these conceptual models in the spaces of the real and hence remodel space itself'" (Rose 1999: 37). The concept of modelling establishes a relation between abstract models of space and local place. Translation has a similar analytic function to modelling in that it examines " . . . the alliances . . . forged between the objectives of authorities wishing to govern and the personal projects of those organizations, groups and individuals who are the subjects of government" (Rose 1999: 48). Among historians of the present reference to translation occurs at the limits of the Foucauldian problem-space in order to think linkages between truthful expertise and social practice.

The grafting of actor–network theory onto the history of the present has proved to be intellectually productive, but it does not work particularly well for our purposes. Our research site centrally poses questions about the relation of public health knowledge to law and to the political. As we have noted, reporting a case of a notifiable infectious disease to WHO was in the second half of the 20th century a sovereign act under international public health law. Global emergency vigilance required not simply a change in the practices of public health expertise, but also a change in juridical right and political power beyond the sovereign; that is, emergency vigilance implicates world order. The relation between the scientific and the political/legal is arguably the weakest part of actor–network theory, which centers explanation on the laboratory where scientists are theorized as creating hybrids that combine scientific signs and material processes, that is, material–semiotic hybrids like thyroid stimulating hormone (TSH) or DNA (Callon 1994, 2001; Latour 1987). Once formed, these hybrids pass into expansive translation networks that comprise many interested social actors, including at a limit those who fund research and development (Latour 1987: 167–173). In principle, scientific networks might be extended to link with the political and the legal conceived as actors in a network of alliances. The political and the legal would then come to science from without at the end of the translation network. It should be noted that Latour turned to the topic of science and the political in *We Have Never Been Modern* (1993) to encourage recognition and debate about the effects of science by conceptualizing the place of proliferating scientific material–semiotic objects within the political.

The actor–network formulation of the relation between science and the political is science centered and does not examine the specificity of law and the political in their difference from science. The political and the legal should not be theorized as one among many social actors as this elides the distinction between fundamentally different orders of knowledge with attendant power effects. Devalorization and misrecognition of nonscientific knowledge is characteristic of our present, and social scientists might well be interested in the political and in juridical right as knowledge forms that constitute common fates and shared worlds, not through material–semiotic hybrids, but through symbolic processes. We return to this discussion in Chapter 5.

Our focus on global public health harmonizes with a broadening of Foucauldian work on health, particularly in the field of anthropology, beyond its recent research trajectory in human genetics. Public health does not reduce life to the gene; epidemiology has a robust conception of population; ecological studies form a growth area in public health expertise. This book seeks to revitalize an older research interest among historians of the present in public health. Foucault's own writings frequently dealt with public health. The famous "Panopticism" chapter of *Discipline and Punish* (Foucault 1975/1979: 195–199) begins with an analysis of measures taken against the plague in late 17th century French towns. In the midst of a book remembered for its contributions to theorizing the history of punishment and the prison, Foucault analyzed the public health measures found for several centuries in Europe prior to the sanitary measures of the mid-19th century, calling these "a compact model of the disciplinary mechanism" for training the bodies of individuals in factories, schools, barracks, hospitals, and prisons. In Foucault's 1979 article "The Politics of Health in the Eighteenth Century" (Foucault 1979/1997: 90–91), he suggested that medicine had historically been two-sided, one side being oriented to care of individual patients and the laws of the market, the other concerned with collective health and disease as social and political problems. The public health side of medicine received more expansive treatment in Foucault's 1975–1976 and 1977–1978 lectures at the Collège de France (Foucault 2003, 2007) where he investigated the historical formation of public health measures that sought to improve the health of population by acting on birth rates, mortality rates, illness, accidents, injuries, and so forth. Foucault's analyses often examined the history of infectious disease control. This aspect of Foucault's work has been taken up in some of the writings of François Delaporte, most particularly *Disease and Civilization: The Cholera in Paris, 1832* (Delaporte 1986), although the deeper influence on Delaporte's writing has been the historian and philosopher Georges Canguilhem.

Recent work by Stephen J. Collier, Andrew Lakoff, and Paul Rabinow (Collier, Lakoff, & Rabinow 2004; Lakoff 2006; Collier & Lakoff 2006) at the Berkeley Center for the Anthropology of the Contemporary (University of California) has begun to investigate biosecurity from a broadly Foucauldian perspective. Their research pertains to the USA and does not take up questions of infectious disease, public health, and global biopolitics, our problematic here. We note that our analysis of global emergency vigilance differs from the theorization of "preparedness" and "population security" found in Collier and Lakoff's preliminary studies. Collier and Lakoff (2006) theorize preparedness as a practice aiming to conserve political and economic infrastructure, arguing it has displaced practices oriented to conserving the health of population. Given that public health today remains a practice oriented to the health of population, and concepts of population are found throughout contemporary biomedical research from clinical trials to cohort studies, population remains a highly significant concept within the contemporary health sciences and medical reasoning. Global emergency vigilance does not displace the population concept.

Our work on emergency vigilance is in part intended as a contribution to Foucauldian work on biopolitics, specifically global biopolitics. We take "biopolitics" in Foucault's (2007: 1) original sense as a terrain that was precipitated by the 18th century European conception of humanity as a species, a cosmological shift from the prior Christian conception of humanity as the hinge between heaven and earth. This cosmological shift was the precondition for the projects that acted to link humans as biological beings with politics and power strategies. Biopolitics has a defining objective: optimizing the human species at the level of its life and health. However, biopolitical projects act, not on the human species in general, but on human collectivities (e.g., citizens of states, peoples), abstract aggregates (e.g., populations), and the bodies of persons variously partitioned by nation, ethnicity, gender, and social class (among other divisions). Global emergency vigilance may be understood as biopolitical because it acts to stabilize national and international economies and political regimes against the effects of epidemics and disasters.

The study of biopolitics has for the most part been nationally focused, although recently there has been growing interest in the global pharmaceutical industry (Petryna, Lakoff, & Kleinman 2006) and global sociotechnical networks (Ong & Collier 2005). As our work has examined public health above the level of the nation, this book concerns what the historian Alison Bashford has called "global biopolitics" (2006: 67). Bashford introduced the term global biopolitics to conceptualize "the history of biopolitics beyond the nation" (2006: 67, 81) in contrast to Mitchell Dean's "international biopolitics" (Dean 1999: 100), which occurs in the space between sovereign states. Bashford formulated the concept of global biopolitics in the context of examining what was called 'world health' programming at the League of Nations between World Wars I and II, arguing that global biopolitics in this period was focused on population management through hygiene.

Emergency vigilance within contemporary global biopolitics is a very different form of reasoning and technical intervention than that of world health in the 1920s and 1930s. Whereas world health sought to improve international health through hygiene, the global biopolitics we are examining aims at the containment of international emergencies through very early warning and response. Unlike hygiene, emergency vigilance is about control rather than prevention. As a biopolitical project, emergency vigilance marked a revision of infectious disease and disaster management as a concern of the North as well as the South. During the second half of the 20th century, infectious disease control in international public health policy had primarily been viewed as a problem of the South, a problem given the remedy of what was called development. The rationale for and operation of emergency vigilance, however, is not articulated to development economics.

The ascendance of emergency vigilance as a programmatic form of international public health action was due to the political forces that backed it in a world regionally divided between North and South: global biopolitics. Emergency vigilance is global in the additional sense of having constituted a new level of political power in global biopolitics. The formation of a world on alert transformed international health law and politics, giving WHO authorized powers to know about global public health emergencies independently of sovereign power and to publicize emergencies, if necessary in the absence of sovereign consent.

C) Studies in the Social Organization of Knowledge

Our research site raised questions about politically and legally mandated courses of action in disease and emergency reporting. It also invited us to think about the relations between official and unofficial knowledge of outbreak, the conversion of news into verified knowledge, and more generally, global emergency vigilance as an apparatus coordinating disparate knowledge relations. The combination of our prior interest in the social organization of knowledge and the complex knowledge relations of international public health led us to link the history of the present with studies in the social organization of knowledge.

'Studies in the social organization of knowledge' is a term used to refer to a trajectory of sociological research on 'ruling relations' inspired by the work of Dorothy Smith (1974a, 1974b, 1987, 1990a, 1990b, 1999, 2005). Smith's early writings were produced as part of a body of North American second-wave feminist scholarship that critiqued the presumed objectivity of the social and natural sciences. Smith's distinctive contributions were her critique of sociology as an objectifying discourse and her formulation of an alternative sociological project that took the standpoint of the 'everyday' as the point of departure for empirical inquiry into the social relations that shape, limit, and organize experience. Building on feminist methods of consciousness raising, Smith argued that the standard conceptual practices of established sociology obscured people's experiences, "transposing the actualities of [their] lives . . . into the conceptual currency with which [they] can be governed" (D. Smith 1974a: 8). Smith's alternative was to begin sociological inquiry in the local particularities of people's everyday lives rather than the formal categories of sociological discourse, with the goal of exploring how those particularities are geared into extended social and institutional relations.

Smith's sociology is distinguished from other successor projects with similar historical roots in that its analytic preoccupation is not the discovery of

meaning, the description of sympathetic accounts of experience, or the reha-
bilitation of rationality through attention to emotion. Rather, its analytic
object is the ruling relations, conceived of by Smith as a historically specific
mode of social organization characteristic of advanced capitalist societies.
Extending Marx's analysis of the early capitalist economy as a "specialized
organization of relations of dependence" (D. Smith 1999: 77), Smith conceived of the ruling relations analogously as an organization of consciousness and agency that stands apart from the local and particular. The ruling
relations involve a complex of administrative, managerial, and professional
practices and discourses that govern contemporary society. They are per-
vasively interconnected, extend beyond the state as the locus of power, and
coordinate people in the "sites of their bodily being into relations operating
independently of person, place and time" (D. Smith 1999: 75).

One of the most significant contributions of Smith's sociology is its treatment of texts as the central medium of ruling relations; the latter are inher-
ently text-mediated forms of social organization. In studies of the social
organization of knowledge, texts are treated as the bridge between local
sites of embodied activity and translocal, abstracted ruling relations. They
are fundamental to the production and circulation of objectified forms of
discourse upon which translocal forms of coordination rely. Smith introduced a distinctively sociological treatment of texts within the empirical
exploration of contemporary forms of ruling discourse, one in which texts
are analyzed not for surface meaning alone but are explored in 'action.'
Texts are investigated ethnographically as material objects with a standard
replicable form that, when engaged by particular readers, enter their local
activities into forms of organization that extend across time and place.

Smith's invitation to produce an alternative sociology that investigates
extended forms of coordination and control that "are not wholly knowable
from within the scope of local experience" (McCoy 2008: 701) has been
taken up by researchers both within and beyond sociology. A range of studies exploring the text-mediated forms of knowledge organizing relations
within and across health care (Mykhalovskiy 2008, 2003; Diamond 1992;
Rankin & Campbell 2006), education (Griffith & D. Smith 2005), policing
(G. Smith 1998), accounting (McCoy 1998), housing (Luken & Vaughan
2006), multiculturalism and immigration (Ng 1990, 1995), and other sites
of professional work and discourse has been conducted by sociologists,
health researchers, social workers, and education researchers, amongst
others.

The approach taken to the social organization of knowledge in these
studies typically emphasizes the textual mechanics of objectification
through which the particular and local are transformed into governable
form. But studies in the social organization of knowledge are also animated
by a broader spirit of empirical investigation often expressed in colloquial
form as 'how things work' or 'how things are put together.' The pairing
of a concern with 'how things work' with the investigation of the play of

knowledge in translocal relations distinguishes studies in the social organization of knowledge from work inspired by social construction of knowledge traditions. The latter animate inquiry with an understanding that all knowledge is socially created and therefore value laden, situated, and partial. Studies in the social organization of knowledge, by contrast, privilege how knowledge 'works' by posing questions about how knowledge operates as an active constituent of the social, shaping how things get done and enabling characteristic forms of social relations. It is this feature of this body of work's analytic orientation to knowledge that has most influenced our own investigation.

D) A Dialogue

The dialogue between the history of the present and studies in the social organization of knowledge that we have produced shapes the analysis we offer in this book in a number of ways. For example, the notion of the 'active concept,' used in Chapter 2, is a joint product of studies in the social organization of knowledge and the history of the present. The active concept owes much to Dorothy Smith's (1990a, 1990b) theorization of the "active text" as a constituent of public discourse. The active text is an "institutional account" that produces state activities as mandated, reconstructing and subsuming the accounts of eyewitnesses (D. Smith 1990a: 152–153). We have transposed Smith's active text to the level of the concept. Our treatment of the 'active concept' is consonant with Foucauldian work on the historical formation of concepts (Foucault 1976: 56–63), which follows in the tradition of the historical epistemology of science in giving primacy to concepts as definitive of modern science.

Our analysis in Chapter 3 of unofficial knowledge sourced primarily in news is an unusual empirical site for both schools. The examination of news differs from standard Foucauldian work in dealing with knowledge that does not belong to expertise; news is neither a theoretical knowledge (*savoir*) nor a science (*connaissance*). Moreover, our focus is on the effects of unofficial news on public health *connaissance*. News is also an unusual focus for studies in the social organization of knowledge, the formative contributions of which explore the social organization of administrative facticity by analyzing the mechanics of standardized administrative texts such as intake forms. Still, the interest in textual practices on the part of studies in the social organization of knowledge directs our attention to innovations introduced by GPHIN (the early warning online detection and alert system) in the automated processes for searching and identifying relevant electronic text information from the colossus of global online news. From a studies in the social organization of knowledge perspective, early warning outbreak detection and alert is, in part, a sequence of practices through which information produced as part of the social organization of news consumption is identified, modified, verified, and attached to the relevancies of global public health where it coordinates new relations of vigilance.

Finally, our analysis of the introduction of the concept of "events that may constitute a public health emergency of international concern" in the IHR (2005) and its operationalization by an algorithm and guide draws on both the history of the present and studies in the social organization of knowledge. Our analysis is Foucauldian in that it is both historical and discursive. But there is a second aspect that belongs to studies in the social organization of knowledge. While we have not explored how the algorithm and guide have been activated by actual readers, as a strict studies in the social organization of knowledge approach would require, our analysis treats the algorithm and guide as textual devices that introduce new forms of public health reasoning into the field and that seek to standardize and coordinate the judgement of local public health officials.

The collaboration between studies in the history of the present and the social organization of knowledge through which we have written this book enables the history of the present to ask questions about how the rational schemas of truthful expertise enter into institutions, social relations, and social processes. This facilitates inquiries about what Foucault's work refused: the distribution and effects of a discourse at the level of social relations. Studies in the social organization of knowledge encourages analysis of knowledge forms beyond those that have been stabilized in the rare and repeatable discourse of the archive. This expanded conception of knowledge includes the abstract discourses of expertise, everyday knowledge and, for our purposes, the mass media.

The dialogue we have constructed between the history of the present and studies in the social organization of knowledge has a number of characteristics. We have used the history of the present and the social organization of knowledge to extend each other, moving from historical description and flat discourse analysis to the social analysis of knowledge relations. Foucauldian analytics are thus given an exterior, as is studies in the social organization of knowledge. The idea of the active concept provides a point of articulation between the internal textual analysis and historical description found in the history of the present and the analysis of the transformative effect of a concept on institutional relations. Our treatment of outbreak detection is centered on a social organization of knowledge analysis of the changing institutional relations between official and unofficial information of outbreak. The terms of the analysis are in part set by a Foucauldian distinction between truthful knowledge, here reports based on clinical and laboratory diagnoses and news. Medical knowledge is thus given an outside, a politically and legally consequential outside. In our analysis of international public health law, the analytics alternate. Our analysis of the problematization of the IHR is animated by the history of the present while our discussion of the novel text-mediated forms of public health reasoning and practice projected by the IHR and their list and algorithm proceeds in a manner consistent with studies in the social organization of knowledge. Each school has been left in its distinctiveness at the level of theory, with no attempt to construct a synthesis: a relation of dialogue.

Research Design

Our research design required historical and contemporary sources in order to compare the knowledge relations of international public health before and after the invention of emergency vigilance. Our methodology combined key informant interviews with archival and document research. In order to understand the social organization of knowledge in emergency vigilance, we elected to do onsite interviews that also provided an element, albeit small, of ethnographic method.

The participants in our interviews were public health personnel who have been central to the development of global emergency vigilance. An additional two participants were members of a news service. With the exception of one telephone interview, all key informant interviews took place in Geneva (Switzerland), Ottawa (Canada), and Toronto (Canada). All interviews were recorded and later transcribed. On July 26 and 27, 2004, we interviewed 10 managers and staff of the Global Public Health Intelligence Network (GPHIN). The onsite GPHIN interviews took place at the Centre for Emergency Preparedness and Response, Public Health Agency of Canada, Ottawa. (The Public Health Agency of Canada is part of the Canadian federal government.) We additionally consulted GPHIN in early 2009 to update and check the accuracy of our comments on the organization of their work. Two further onsite interviews were conducted in May 2005 with personnel at a global news service that provides online information to GPHIN. One research participant was interviewed by telephone; this participant was associated with ProMED-mail, the first of the online early warning outbreak detection systems.

In September 2005 we interviewed one research participant at WHO headquarters in Geneva. We returned to WHO headquarters in September through October 2006 to conduct interviews with 6 additional members of WHO. At this time we reinterviewed the WHO research participant who had spoken with us in 2005, bringing the total number of interviewees at WHO headquarters during 2006 to 7. The interviews ranged from 60 to 120 minutes. In order to protect personal confidentiality, we have chosen to identify research participants collectively in our text as 'GPHIN Interview' and 'WHO Interview.' For the protection of the personal confidentiality of those interviewed at the global news service provider, we elected not to quote from the interviews here.

When we presented work in progress at conferences, historians rankled at our claims that online early warning outbreak detection and alert represented anything historically new. Although we realize this is an irresistible stance for historians in the presence of sociologists, we reflected on our position and decided we had been reproducing the viewpoint of our sources and research participants in emphasizing the worth of their work by contrast to an oversimplified past. As a result of the historians' intervention we decided that more careful comparison of outbreak detection and the previous form of epidemiological surveillance was needed, leading us to undertake 4 weeks of research at the Archives of the World Health Organization in Geneva. Our archival research investigated epidemiological surveillance at WHO from 1946 through 1986, that is, from its founding to the latest possible date we were able to obtain files subject to the usual 20-year rule; the earliest available archival records that were available to us were organizational documents from 20 years prior to our research date. Our primary focus in this archival research was on the relation between official and unofficial report of outbreak/epidemic. We also examined unpublished WHO documents pertaining to the history of epidemiological surveillance. Although we have in the present chapter argued that a rupture in epidemiological surveillance methods did occur at the turn of the 21st century, we have done so by more careful comparison of emergency vigilance with epidemiological communications in the second half of the 20th century at WHO.

The effect of reflecting on contemporary history by using a mixed methodology of archival, document, and interview research is to bring past and present very close together: an historicized present. The present gains a prearchival quality as a locus that works on and revises the stable, circular impasses of international public health in the second half of the 20th century. The combination of empirical methods gives this book a genealogical character, although it is a very recent genealogy of how emergencies come into public health knowledge.

2   Emerging Infectious Diseases
An Active Concept

This chapter provides a short history (between 1989 and 1996) of the emerging infectious diseases (EID) concept from its formulation in the USA to its arrival at WHO. Our historical discussion treats EID as an 'active' concept, one that altered understandings of infectious disease in ways that mobilized widespread public health concern over new microbial threats and drove significant institutional change in the scope and form of global public health surveillance and field response.

The phenomenal success of the EID concept has been discussed in popular and scholarly sources. For example, a number of popular histories of the formation of the concept in the U.S. context have been written. Some, such as Garrett's *The Coming Plague: Newly Emerging Diseases in a World Out of Balance* (1994) and Henig's *A Dancing Matrix: Voyages Along the Viral Frontier* (1993), offer predictable narratives of heroic scientific struggle against a new brand of dangerous and relentless viruses and microbes. Popular accounts tell of the menacing threat EID presents to humanity, recapitulating a story originally formulated by those who invented the EID concept as a call to arms for reinvigorating political and public health interest in infectious disease control.

Others have written more critically about EID. Among the most prominent of these authors is noted physician and anthropologist Paul Farmer (1999) whose work has focused on tuberculosis in Haiti. Farmer treats the EID concept as inappropriate for the analysis of global public health, asking "[i]f certain populations have long been afflicted by these disorders, why are the diseases considered 'new' or 'emerging'?" (Farmer 1999: 39). There is nothing new, emerging, or re-emerging about tuberculosis in Haiti. Farmer argues that because tuberculosis is the world's leading cause of death from infectious diseases, and that because most of these deaths are in the global South and among the poor in the global North, to call tuberculosis "new" or "emerging" is implicitly to perceive its history from the perspective of the rich and to value human life in the global North above that in the global South (Farmer 1999: 57, 185). A second critical perspective is found in the work of the historian Nicholas King (2001, 2002) who has written about EID from a history of science perspective. King (2001:16) conceptualizes EID as a civic advocacy campaign that began in an alliance of U.S. virologists, epidemiologists, molecular biologists, and public health officials. The EID campaign was, King holds, primarily about corporate profit: "the global circulation of medical products" (2002: 779) and the marketing of films and books in consumer culture.

Our analysis of EID differs from the existing literature in a number of ways. While we are sympathetic to Farmer's critique of EID and later address the implications of EID for public health priorities in the global South, ours is not a normative treatment of the concept. Rather, we approach EID as an object for a sociological analysis of public health knowledge. We are interested in exploring EID not simply along a good/bad axis but in terms of its effectivity as a concept and the social relations that it coordinates. This stance involves taking some distance from the pure critique of EID and most certainly from the more common position of popularizing the concept through endless discussion of its threat to human health. It also requires a departure from King's commodity economic explanations of the EID concept against which we would emphasize EID as a transformation in public health governance.

As sociologists, our interest is in EID as an active concept, one that has provoked far-reaching legal, political, and technical transformations in international communicable disease control. As many have noted, EID was formulated in the context of U.S. debates about domestic and international infectious disease control that problematized popular, medical, and political understandings of infectious disease as a concern that had, for all practical purposes, been solved within U.S. public health in the 1960s after the conclusion of the polio epidemic. The EID concept amounted to a rebranding of infectious diseases, heightening their political and economic profile after decades of neglect and indifference in the global North. We argue that the invention of the EID concept shifted established understandings of infectious disease in two interconnected ways. First, EID brought into discourse a new order of threat to human health: previously unknown infectious diseases or known diseases whose incidence is increasing. The EID concept broke with dominant U.S. public health assumptions that for all practical purposes bacteria and viruses were unchanging, static entities. The inventors of the EID concept linked molecular biology and ecological studies with public health, emphasizing that bacteria and viruses have the capacity to be genetically flexible, a capacity that had profound practical implications for public health systems. Second, EID formulated such infectious diseases geopolitically as phenomena that threatened U.S. national security. EID thus powerfully called into question existing national and international infectious disease control arrangements.

Disconnecting the USA from international microbial threats would require a far faster knowledge of local outbreaks by international public health authorities, necessitating the speeding up of surveillance data, the subordination of local historical time to synchronized world time, and the opening of local place to continuous global spatial relations. The

EID concept problematized the spatial and temporal relations of international communicable disease surveillance at WHO. Responding to U.S.-led demands for dealing with EID, WHO developed a new strategic plan that set a new standard in international infectious disease control: the world on alert.

Our interest in the contextualization of EID has been provoked by the work of the anthropologist Marilyn Strathern (1999) whose work on recent technologies of procreation such as in vitro fertilization (IVF) has investigated the significance of context for rendering ideas and statements intelligible. She has theorized the global as an emergent context constituted in part from the occlusion of its social, political, economic, and cultural dimensions together with the formation of new universal practices and standards that fashion particular types of connections. In the case of global public health, we are dealing with what Strathern (1999: 187) has termed an "order of knowledge" that has a politically organized internal division of spatialized contexts. The epistemological shift that EID represents ultimately succeeded in bypassing formal sovereign control of infectious disease report, emancipating public health knowledge of outbreak and other emergencies, and constituting new universal norms and practices for knowing and acting on EID: a global emergency vigilance apparatus that presented EID control as a universal health need, thereby occluding its own context.

We begin by tracing the EID concept from its beginnings in the USA to its reception and reformulation at WHO as a matter of global health. Our account differs from the existent U.S.-focused literature in documenting and analyzing the internationalization of the EID concept in its movement from the USA to global public health at the WHO. We trace the internationalization of the EID concept through a careful reading of a series of policy reports that lead from the Institute of Medicine's (1992) landmark *Emerging Infections: Microbial Threats to Health in the United States* to the U.S.–Canadian alliance forged around EID during 1993 (Lac Tremblant Declaration 1994),[1] followed by the reception of the EID concept at WHO in 1994 and 1995 (WHO 1994, 1995), and ending with the WHO strategic plan, "Emerging and other Communicable Diseases" (WHO 1996). We then turn to two North–South power/knowledge effects associated with the EID concept, the first that renders EID an unstable concept and the second that constitutes EID as a priority of international development assistance for health.

Inventing a Disease Concept

It is conventional to state that public health authorities in the global North during the period from roughly 1960 to 1990 believed that chronic disease had displaced infectious disease as the primary cause of mortality in what was called the "epidemiological transition" (Tulchinsky & Varavikova

2000: 42–43). The nations of the global South were conceptualized as not having passed through this transition. A combination of better nutrition, improved housing, vaccines, antibiotics, and DDT had displaced communicable disease prevention and control as the core activity of public health systems in the global North, although infectious disease was acknowledged by public health authorities as significant within marginalized populations and collectivities, for instance tuberculosis among Aboriginal peoples in Canada and the USA. From the early 1980s the HIV/AIDS pandemic troubled this public health understanding of the health transition, but HIV/AIDS was treated as an exception in health funding and administration, and it is difficult to generalize from what has been constituted as exceptional.

In retrospect it appears that there was a curious lack of integration between bacteriological genetics and public health knowledge during the period from 1950 to 1990, although there did exist minority positions linking the two fields without policy effect. Richard Krause published *The Restless Tide: The Persistent Challenge of the Microbial World* in 1981 when he was Director of the (U.S.) National Institute of Allergy and Infectious Diseases. In it he warned that the USA might face infectious disease epidemics from diverse causes: genetic drift in the microbial world, antibiotic resistance, and social changes related to commerce, agriculture, lifestyle, and war.

Krause's arguments from genetic drift and antibiotic resistance were based on Joshua Lederberg's influential research in bacterial genetics. Lederberg's work of the late 1940s and 1950s decisively showed that bacteria could adapt and evolve quickly. His research proved that bacteria do not simply reproduce themselves identically. The bacterium *Escherichia coli* has a sexual phase during which genetic information is exchanged (conjugation) and bacteriophages transfer genetic information across *Salmonella* bacteria (transduction). The latter process, transduction, explained how bacteria could develop resistance to an antibiotic. The resulting perception of bacteria as genetically flexible was at variance with U.S. public health policy in the second half of the 20th century, which implicitly assumed an unchanging microbial world. Lederberg's research achieved international renown when he shared half the Nobel Prize in 1958,[2] a form of recognition that makes all the more puzzling the decades-long gap between bacterial genetics and public health thinking.

It was during Lederberg's tenure as President of the Rockefeller University (New York City) that opposition crystallized to U.S. public health policy on infectious disease prevention and control. At a university reception held in 1988, Lederberg made casual conversation about infectious diseases with Stephen Morse, a virologist and assistant professor at Rockefeller University (Garrett 1994: 5; Henig 1993: 13). Morse seized upon the opportunity to work with Lederberg, and they formed an alliance, mobilizing like-minded scientists to participate in "Emerging Viruses: The Evolution of Viruses and Viral Diseases," a conference held in Washington, D.C., in May 1989. Chaired by Stephen Morse, the conference was cosponsored by the National Institutes of Health (NIH) and the Rockefeller University (Morse 1993c: xi). It was attended by 200 participants, many of them senior scientists and public health officials such as Donald Henderson (Associate Director for Life Sciences, Office of Science and Technology Policy, Executive Office of the President), Richard Krause (Fogarty International Center, NIH), and Robert E. Shope (Director, Arbovirus Research, Yale University). In his convening speech, Lederberg directed attention to antimicrobial strains of diseases and to infectious diseases, such as HIV/AIDS and Ebola, which were new to the United States (King 2002: 766–767).

The effects of the 1989 Emerging Viruses Conference reached into popular culture and public health policy. The historian Nicholas King (2002: 768–770) has demonstrated that this conference received extensive popular coverage in science news publications by eminent science journalists such as Lawrence Altman (*The New York Times*) and Laurie Garrett (*Newsday*). Scholars in cultural studies and journalism (Moeller 1999; Stabile 1997; Wald 2008) have examined the fascination with infectious disease outbreaks that characterized news, films, and novels from the early 1990s to the present, particularly the novels and subsequent films of the science journalist Richard Preston (*The Hot Zone* [1995] and *The Cobra Event* [1997]). Our own concern, however, lies with the trajectory of the EID concept in public health knowledge rather than in popular culture.

The 1989 Emerging Viruses Conference precipitated a study proposal to the Institute of Medicine (IOM), which was approved in 1989. (The Institute of Medicine is one of four nongovernmental, not-for-profit United States National Academies; its purpose is to provide the U.S. federal government with advice on matters related to medicine, the life sciences, and health.) Consequently, in 1991 an IOM Committee on Emerging Microbial Threats to Health was formed to study emerging infectious diseases and make recommendations about how the U.S. public health system was to prevent and contain them (Lederberg & Shope 1992: vi). The IOM committee, which was co-chaired by Joshua Lederberg and Robert Shope, included Stephen Morse as a member. Its report, *Emerging Infections: Microbial Threats to Health in the United States* (IOM 1992), was published in 1992, appearing a year prior to the collection *Emerging Viruses* (Morse 1993a) that followed Morse's 1989 conference.

Emerging Viruses and *Emerging Infections* formulated a new programme for public health governance that drew on accepted science in microbiology and molecular genetics. In both *Emerging Viruses* and *Emerging Infections* microbes are understood as genetically mutable rather than as fixed entities. From its inception the EID concept has been conceptually coordinated with contemporary genetic approaches to microbiology and molecular biology, aligning public health thinking and practice with genetic knowledge. As a disease concept EID formulates the emergence of microbial entities in genetic terms, transformations posited at the level of microbial being (IOM

1992: 84–105). But it is important to emphasize that EID is also conceived of ecologically. *Emerging Viruses* and *Emerging Infections* are replete with ecological discourse that is drawn upon to think through the conditions of emergence of infectious diseases. Microbial adaptation and change appears as only one of six main factors in disease emergence in the 1992 IOM report; the others focus on ecological factors such as changes in land use and population growth.

The EID concept in *Emerging Viruses* and *Emerging Infections* is conceptually coordinated with U.S. national interests. These works portray the USA as vulnerable to infectious disease in a world represented as increasingly interconnected economically, socially, and microbiologically. Richard Krause begins the "Foreword" to *Emerging Viruses* by noting that "[l]ike science, emerging viruses know no country. There are no barriers to prevent their migration across international boundaries or around the 24 time zones" (Krause 1993: xvii). Lederberg and Shope's "Preface" to *Emerging Infections* also starts with a statement about connectedness: "As the human immunodeficiency virus (HIV) disease pandemic surely should have taught us, in the context of infectious diseases, there is nowhere in the world from which we are remote and no one from whom we are disconnected" (Lederberg & Shope 1992: v). The "we" in this sentence is part of a political language clarified in the next sentence as referring to the USA: "Consequently, some infectious diseases that now affect people in other parts of the world represent potential threats to the United States, because of global interdependence, modern transportation, trade, and changing social and cultural patterns'" (Lederberg & Shope 1992: v). Both *Emerging Viruses* and *Emerging Infections* open with a problematic of connectedness: specifically, how to maintain international connectedness while disconnecting a particular nation from infectious disease spread. The HIV/AIDS pandemic appears in these texts as the paradigmatic contemporary example of the problematic of connectedness (IOM 1992: v; Lederberg 1993: 3; Morse 1993b: 10).

The outcomes of badly governed microbial connectedness are sometimes depicted hyperbolically in *Emerging Viruses* and *Emerging Infections*, particularly by Lederberg, who after referring to the introduction of the myxoma virus that killed 80% of rabbits in Australia, asks rhetorically about what would happen to humans under such conditions: "whether human society could survive left on the beach with only a few percent of survivors. Could they function at any level of culture higher than that of rabbits?" (Lederberg 1993: 8). References to "threats" and the attendant importance of mobilizing against threats are found throughout the 1992 IOM report, appearing as early as its subtitle, "microbial threats to health in the United States." The conception of nature itself as vengeful and threatening is also present in *Emerging Viruses* and *Emerging Infections* and was reported in the mass media depictions of epidemic as nature's revenge on humanity in, for instance, Richard Preston's novel *The Hot Zone* (Stabile 1997).

We note in passing that although medicine cannot function without the distinction between health and sickness—that is, without a concept of the normal and the pathological—the notion of microbes as inevitably threatening is clearly partial, for, in microbiological terms, without microbes there would be no decomposition; without decomposition there would be no soil; without soil there would be no plants; and without plants there would be no food. Many microbes might appear to be our good friends, and indeed the political distinction between friend and enemy functions badly for understanding the relation between the human world and the microbial world, though the distinction provides bountiful social and cultural effects.

Emerging Viruses and *Emerging Infections* present the dilemmas of global interconnectedness as new to the late 20th century, understanding the speed and numbers of people travelling internationally to have created historically novel conditions for infectious disease spread. However, this theme has been part of international public health discussions since the first International Sanitary Conference in Paris during 1851. The historian François Delaporte (1986: 189–195) treats the 1851 International Sanitary Conference as marking the end of European practices that since the early modern period had dealt with plague through quarantine and *cordons sanitaires*, exclusively disciplinary solutions to the problems of infectious disease transmission that failed in the European cholera outbreak of 1832. The International Sanitary Conferences (1851–1894), which resulted in the first international law dealing with infectious diseases control, framed discussion in terms of a "shrinking and boundless world" (Huber 2006: 455). The public health problematic of preventing international disease transmission while simultaneously preserving international migration, trade, and transportation has framed the terms of international public health policy since 1851.[3] The perception of the present moment as one of unprecedented novelty has also characterized international public health discussions since that time.

Morse's edited collection and the 1992 IOM report introduced disease concepts that were announced in the titles of the two books: emerging viruses and emerging infections. For the virologist Morse, "emerging viruses" referred to "viruses that either have newly appeared in the population or are rapidly expanding their range, with a corresponding increase in cases of disease" (Morse 1993b: 10). Because many infectious diseases are not considered viral, the IOM report replaced "viruses" with "infections" but retained "emerging" to produce the concept "emerging infections" and/ or "new and emerging infectious diseases." In the words of Lederberg and Shope, "[a]lthough the conference [Morse's 1989 Emerging Viruses Conference] focused on viruses; it spurred interest in the emergence and resurgence of *all* classes of infectious agents" (emphasis in original; Lederberg & Shope 1992: v). The IOM report thus defined the concept of emerging infectious diseases more broadly than Morse had defined the concept of "emerging viruses." Emerging infectious diseases consist of all those "clini-cally distinct conditions whose incidence in humans has increased" (IOM 1992: 34). As incidence in an epidemiological sense may only be estimated for a defined population over a specific period of time, the committee speci-fied that its work had "focused on diseases that have emerged in the United States within the past two decades" (IOM 1992: 34). The logical implica-tion of the IOM's definition of EID is that it will vary according to context, that is, the EID list for the USA may not necessarily be identical to the list for France, Mexico, or Sri Lanka.

Applied to the USA, the EID concept unified previously disparate phe-nomena, linking diseases newly introduced to the USA from elsewhere (e.g., HIV/AIDS, dengue), diseases whose incidence had previously declined called "re-emerging" (e.g., tuberculosis), infectious diseases previously present domestically but whose incidence had increased (e.g., Lyme disease), and known conditions now thought to be caused by microbes (e.g., peptic ulcers). As a concept EID produced a broad problem-space for public health action, mobilizing against "complacency" by emphasizing the growing number of infectious diseases with increasing incidence rates within the USA.

Emerging Infections was more specifically innovative in its ecologi-cal classification of infectious diseases, relating disease transmission to socioeconomic change rather than to a classification of agents (viral, bac-terial, and others). Close to half the IOM report analyzed ecological fac-tors that contribute to disease emergence, and it explained how humans and microbes are multifariously connected through land use and economic change, increases in international travel and commercial activity, public health collapse, and human population change and behavior.

Emerging Infections and *Emerging Viruses* were oriented to preserving health in the USA, portraying the global South as a source of infectious disease threat. Written with a U.S. audience in mind, both reports recom-mended strengthening domestic surveillance and preparedness to address EID containment. Each report also called for the establishment of new global surveillance mechanisms, although they were not certain of the insti-tution most appropriate to develop them. David Henderson, former Chief of the Smallpox Eradication Programme at WHO, characterized WHO viral disease programming as underfunded, understaffed, and decentralized, making the CDC (Atlanta, Georgia) the only organization capable of lead-ing international surveillance, with "no option but to acknowledge CDC as an international resource, to fund it appropriately, and to acknowledge its mandate in legislation" (Henderson 1993: 286).[4] Henderson's recom-mendation—a network of research centers headed by the CDC—in effect proposed a return to the epidemiological intelligence of the Euro-American colonial era wherein the colonized had little control over infectious disease report (see Chapter 3 for discussion). Morse's contribution to *Emerging Viruses* followed Henderson in suggesting that a worldwide surveillance and response network be created with combined clinical, diagnostic, and

research centers (Morse 1993b: 21) but differed from Henderson in suggesting that "any network should function in connection with WHO as an
umbrella to establish international cooperation" (Morse 1993a: 22).

Unlike *Emerging Viruses*, which was an academic book edited by a
university professor, *Emerging Infections* as an IOM report was structured to have formal recommendations. These included alterations to
domestic surveillance, clarification of the CDC's role in multilateral surveillance, and a proposal to form a global surveillance network (IOM
1992: 134–137). The impetus for the global surveillance network was
to come from the USA, and perhaps also its directorship: "The committee recommends that the United States take the lead in promoting the
development and implementation of a comprehensive global infectious
disease surveillance system" (IOM 1992: 137). Global surveillance, it was
suggested, would have four components: early detection on the basis of
clinical signs and symptoms; laboratories to identify infectious agents;
information dissemination; a system to respond to agencies and individuals and to mobilize field teams to control outbreaks (IOM 1992: 135). The
IOM conceptualized surveillance as case based, projecting the national
surveillance programme invented under Langmuir at the CDC during
the 1960s (see discussion in Chapter 5) throughout the globe. Despite
ambivalence towards WHO, which is by turns praised for its work on
smallpox and condemned for lacking a mechanism to enforce the terms
of the IHR, *Emerging Infections* recommends that U.S. efforts to form a
global surveillance system be "undertaken through the US representative
to the World Health Assembly" (IOM 1992: 137).

The CDC is the leading U.S. federal institution mandated to deal with
disease control and prevention. Its National Center for Infectious Diseases
(NCID) convened a board meeting in December 1992 to discuss *Emerging
Inflections* (Berkelman & Freeman 2004: 357). The December 1992 meeting recommended that the CDC formulate a response to EID. The CDC
response (written by a group led by Ruth Berkelman, then NCID Deputy
Director) was drafted within a month, although the final version, *Addressing Emerging Infectious Disease Threats: A Prevention Strategy for the
United States* (Centers for Disease Control and Prevention [CDC] 1994)
was not published until April 1994. NCID support for the 1992 IOM report
occurred in the context of a 1993 U.S. federal government directive that
would have cut NCID staff by 358 full time equivalents (FTEs; Berkelman
& Freeman 2004: 358). The NCID did extensive publicity for its proposed
EID prevention strategy and successfully secured national funding for it
in 1994 (Berkelman & Freeman 2004: 363). *Addressing Emerging Infectious Disease Threats* responded to the IOM report with detailed policy
recommendations for its implementation. In it the CDC put further pressure on WHO to strengthen its global surveillance activities and suggested
that a global consortium of research centers for detecting, monitoring, and
investigating emerging infections be established "under the direction of an

international steering committee, possibly chaired by the WHO" (CDC 1994: 21). The CDC report put on record what was already obvious: U.S. public health officials were prepared to move on the global surveillance of EID independent of WHO. Yet the NCID discovered EID surveillance was a rather hard sell with public officials pre-2001, as politicians and bureaucrats did not understand the significance of public health surveillance (Berkelman & Freeman 2004: 385, Ftn. 44).

Emerging Viruses and *Emerging Infections* framed a long-standing U.S. critique of international infectious disease surveillance at WHO in terms of the new urgency of EID control. WHO's capacity to engage in infectious disease surveillance was framed as having gaps and delays. Diseases reportable under the IHR went without notification or delayed notification (IOM 1992: 132). Diagnoses were often not confirmed by laboratories (IOM 1992: 134). Early detection of infectious disease outbreaks, and sometimes of causal agents before the development of symptoms, was called for (IOM 1992: 42). Yet what social, political, and technical form global surveillance was to take lacked clarity in the early 1990s, with many models proposed.

The EID concept was from the first articulated to the protection of U.S. national interests. We have shown that EID specifically formulated infectious diseases as a threat to the USA—a microbial threat to the health of its citizens, its economy, and its global dominance. EID was one of the two targets of early U.S. biosecurity discourse as it was being formulated in the early 1990s, the other target being bioweapons. The invention of the EID concept coincided with the revelation of the extent of the Soviet bioweapons programme, initially in intelligence circles after the 1989 defection and debriefing of the USSR scientist Pasechnik (Hart 2006: 133, 147), and then publicly after the formal Russian declaration in 1992 that the Soviet Union had an offensive bioweapons programme that contravened the Biological and Toxin Weapons Convention to which the former Soviet Union was a signatory (Hart 2006: 150). The result was a securitizing of U.S. domestic public health around two foci: EID and bioweapons.

The two men whose work we have repeatedly cited here, Stephen Morse and Joshua Lederberg, were each instrumental in the formation of early biosecurity concepts and policy. Morse served as the program manager for Biodefense at the Defense Advanced Research Projects Agency (DARPA) in the U.S. Department of Defense between 1996 and 2000.[5] Prior to his work on EID, Lederberg had long been a respected adviser to the U.S. government on science policy (Wright 2007: 67). Susan Wright has documented how Lederberg regarded defense against EID and bioweapons as identical in surveillance terms, each requiring early detection and containment of outbreak plus new therapies (Wright 2007: 73). While we would agree with Nicholas King (2002) that EID was constituted as a U.S. national security matter during the 1990s, we do not characterize this change as being primarily one of integrating infectious disease treatments such as vaccines into international development, but rather with national stability and the continued exercise of sovereign power.

The enormity of the IOM's imaginative achievement in inventing the EID concept can be ascertained by comparing its 1992 report, *Emerging Infections*, with its 1988 report, *The Future of Public Health*. The EID concept gave renewed urgency to communicable disease prevention and control under conditions where *The Future of Public Health* (IOM 1988) aimed more broadly at the renewal of the U.S. public health system. The 1988 report was a major statement of public health needs, but it was not organized around the EID concept. Overall, it argued that the U.S. public health system was in "disarray": "this nation has lost sight of its public health goals and has allowed the system of public health activities to fall into disarray" (IOM 1988: 1). Unlike the 1992 IOM report, *The Future of Public Health* does not exclusively focus on infectious diseases, instead locating infectious disease within a broader public health mandate of present, past, and future crises. Immediate crises included HIV/AIDS and health care for the indigent (IOM 1988: 20–23). The enduring problems for public health comprised injuries, teen pregnancy, control of high blood pressure, smoking, and substance use (IOM 1988: 23–28). Last, "growing challenges" were envisioned as toxic substances and dementias due to Alzheimer's disease or of the Alzheimer's type (IOM 1988: 29–32). The expansiveness of the public health mandate in the 1988 IOM report, an expansiveness typical of public health in the global North in the decades after World War II (Pearce 1996; Susser & Susser 1996), reveals the narrowness of the public health mandate constructed in the 1992 IOM report. *Emerging Infections* was unconcerned with injuries, blood pressure, prenatal care, teen pregnancies, dementias, prenatal care, and chronic diseases not due to infections. *The Future of Public Health* was insightful in calling attention to the political marginalization of public health in the USA, noting that public health tended to be driven by "crises, hot issues, and the concerns of organized interest groups" (IOM 1988: 4). The formulation of the EID concept in the 1992 IOM report made public health into a public problem by concentrating on infectious disease, selecting those whose incidence was increasing. Each of these IOM reports had major policy effects on the U.S. public health system, with the 1992 report having immediate outcomes and the 1988 report longer term ones (Tilson & Berkowitz 2006: 901–02).

A number of general observations about early uses of the EID concept arise here. 'Emerging infectious diseases' forms a collective term that encompasses diverse infectious diseases which, integrated into a single concept, are made into dynamic threats to human health in our present. The EID concept redefines the main goal of communicable disease control, priorizing the emerging over the nonemerging (i.e., those diseases whose incidence is not increasing). The sense of 'emerging' intended by EID applies to diseases previously unknown in humans or previously unknown in a public health jurisdiction and to diseases resurging after their incidence has been reduced.

The concept of emergence is characterized by potentiality; that is, diseases can pass over or not pass over into actuality.[6] In the Aristotelian theory of *dynamis/energeia*, the potential contains unknown possibilities that exceed what exists in the actual. However, not all that is potential passes over into the actual. It is this radical conception of the potential that was linked to public health thinking about infectious diseases in the EID concept. EID precipitated a new standard for infectious disease control: the earliest possible public health knowledge of infectious diseases as their unknowable potential becomes actual. It redefined the target of communicable disease control as responsibility for both known and unknown infectious diseases, actual and potential. The demand on public health surveillance systems is thus not confined to tracking known diseases, but instead extends to identifying the appearance of the previously unknown.

EID coded for and implanted a renewed sense of vulnerability to infectious diseases in the global North. It may be termed a 'perspectival' concept because the increasing incidence of any infectious disease is a judgment made on the basis of comparing current rates with prior rates for a particular population in a particular place. Defined as a rise in the incidence rate of an infectious disease, lists of EIDs must be expected to vary nationally and regionally. It can always be asked of EID, "Emerging for whom and where?" Indeed, as we will show in the final section of this chapter, the EID concept is perspectival in the sense of having no fixed meaning, being continually recontextualized and revised in the global South.

Internationalizing Emerging Infectious Diseases

The 1992 IOM report conceptualized EID as transborder phenomena that threaten U.S. domestic health. It spatialized EID as a problem related to globalization, which thus could not be addressed solely through domestic health measures. Rather than pursue unilateral action, the USA chose international diplomacy to try to persuade allies and international health organizations to develop new measures for controlling the spread of EID. Through this diplomacy the EID concept was internationalized. We document the formation of a U.S.–Canadian alliance in EID control, followed by a series of WHO consultations that put pressure on WHO to deal with the international transmission of EID. The U.S.-led diplomatic efforts met with success as early as 1995 with the formation of a new WHO division, Emerging and Other Communicable Diseases, together with resolutions of the World Health Assembly that called for new efforts in communicable disease control to deal with EID and for the revision of the IHR (1969).

A) The US–Canadian Alliance

Canada was the first international ally to be recruited by the USA in support of its EID strategy. The alliance was formalized at the Workshop on Emerging Infectious Diseases Issues held at Lac Tremblant, Quebec, December 7 through December 9, 1993, 14 months after the IOM report was published in October 1992. The workshop was held to address the 1992 IOM report after discussions at the CDC, WHO, and the Laboratory Centre for Disease Control (LCDC, Ottawa). The report of the 1993 meeting (Lac Tremblant Declaration 1994) was explicitly structured as a Canadian response to the 1992 IOM report, containing sections entitled "The U.S. Institute of Medicine (IOM) Report" (Lac Tremblant Declaration 1994: 3–4), "CDC's Response" (Lac Tremblant Declaration 1994: 7–9), and "The IOM Report: Implications for Canada" (Lac Tremblant Declaration 1994: 14–16).

The Lac Tremblant workshop had 37 Canadian participants and 5 international participants, 3 from the USA and 2 from WHO headquarters in Geneva. Of the 3 U.S. participants, 2 had contributed articles to Morse's *Emerging Viruses*: Dr. C. J. Peters (CDC; Peters et al. 1993) and Dr. Robert Shope (Yale University; Shope & Evans 1993). Shope was also a coeditor of the 1992 IOM report. The third U.S. participant, Dr. Ruth Berkelman, was Deputy Director, National Center for Infectious Diseases, CDC; she had headed the NCID working group that drafted the CDC's response to the IOM report, *Addressing Emerging Infectious Disease Threats: A Prevention Strategy for the United States* (CDC 1994). The two WHO participants consisted of Dr. James LeDuc (Medical Officer, Division of Communicable Diseases) who had also contributed a coauthored article to the Morse collection (LeDuc, Childs, Glass, & Watson 1993) and Dr. Giorgio Torrigiani (Director, Division of Communicable Diseases). Thus, 3 of the 5 international participants at the Lac Tremblant workshop had contributed as authors to the publications that invented the EID concept, *Emerging Viruses* and *Emerging Infections*.

Shope's remarks at the 1993 Lac Tremblant meeting asked that Canada support the USA's proposal for WHO to undertake global EID monitoring: "A Canadian domestic and international plan complimentary to the U.S. response would be mutually reinforcing" (Lac Tremblant Declaration 1994: 4).[7] Acknowledging that most of the IOM's recommendations had been targeted at improving surveillance and response preparedness, Shope justified this focus as due to the unpredictability of EID outbreaks. Mathematics cannot predict future outbreaks, but "[w]hat can be predicted with certainty is that some event will occur; there will be emerging infectious disease problems" (Lac Tremblant Declaration 1994: 4). In Shope's remarks surveillance appears as the primary strategy for EID control and is formulated as a way of governing the certainty of uncertainty.

WHO statements at the Lac Tremblant workshop defined the direction that WHO policy on EID was to take. After noting that communicable diseases had long been recognized as important to public health in the global South, Dr. Torrigiani recommended "a worldwide approach" to deal with communicable diseases, an approach to include "an early warning system" and "an active global surveillance system" (Lac Tremblant Declaration 1994: 5). James LeDuc stated that "WHO is developing a new program for global monitoring of infectious diseases" (Lac Tremblant Declaration 1994: 5) and outlined some of WHO's existing capacity in surveillance, particularly its international networks of collaborating centers.

Ruth Berkelman summarized the CDC's key goals and recommendations that were to appear in its forthcoming report, *Addressing Emerging Infectious Disease Threats* (CDC 1994). The CDC's primary goal was to strengthen domestic and international surveillance of infectious diseases. The second goal of the CDC was to integrate laboratory science and epidemiology into public health (Lac Tremblant Declaration 1994: 8). The latter goal was characteristic of U.S. public health, which since the post-World War II era has led efforts to combine laboratory methods with epidemiology in order to make public health what it considered more scientific (Amsterdamska 2005; Parascandola 1998). Third, the CDC aimed to improve public health communications in relation to practitioners and the public. Last, the CDC proposed that U.S. public health infrastructure and training be renewed at the local, state, and federal levels (Lac Tremblant Declaration 1994: 8). Berkelman also mentioned the proposal for a global consortium of institutions investigating EIDs, although she made no reference to WHO in this regard.

The Canadian understanding at the Lac Tremblant Workshop was that an improved Canadian public health system was being discussed rather than a fundamental rethinking of it. The Canadian presentations at the Lac Tremblant meeting did not focus on EID and for the most part outlined existing domestic surveillance systems, suggesting improvements that might be made to them in order to coordinate jurisdictions, harmonize computer systems, and encourage "cooperation between all groups" (Lac Tremblant Declaration 1994: 13). Such is the culture of Canadian federalism. The need for information sharing and increased resources was repeatedly mentioned. Canadian representatives suggested that advocacy groups along the lines of those that had appeared for HIV/AIDS should be encouraged, and that better linkage between research and infectious disease control was desirable (Lac Tremblant Declaration 1994: 15). No Canadian representative argued EID to be a matter that weakened Canada socially, economically, or politically. Dr. P. Gully, Chief of Sexually Transmitted Diseases, Laboratory Centre for Disease Control (LCDC), raised a fundamental objection to the EID strategy: "There are many 'exotic' diseases that seem remote and of little concern to domestic public health. Should surveillance be preoccupied with remote exotic diseases that might increase over the next decade or focus on conditions that are more common and likely affect the health of a number of Canadians?" (Lac Tremblant Declaration

1994: 11). Gully raised a serious objection to EID strategy and its impact on public health priorities and resource allocation, although he repeated a long Canadian history with his framing of infectious disease found outside Canada as "exotic."

The disjuncture between the Canadian and U.S. presentations had, however, no effect on the two main recommendations of the Lac Tremblant meeting. The leading recommendation endorsed the need for a Canadian national strategy for surveillance and control of EID. The second recommendation suggested a national strategy to improve communications with the public across government departments and to give feedback to those providing EID information (Lac Tremblant Declaration 1994: 18). The third recommendation of the Lac Tremblant consultation had no parallel in other national and international EID reports. It called for an expert group to investigate "ethics and jurisprudence in the area of surveillance and public health interventions" (Lac Tremblant Declaration 1994: 19). That EID strategies might pose ethical and legal questions was not a thought that occurred to authors of the 1992 IOM report, which rested its claims on the self-evidence of promoting health and preventing epidemics. The fourth and final recommendation of the Lac Tremblant Declaration called for sufficient resource allocation to fund primary prevention programmes such as vaccination, with a budget allocation that did not compete with other medical treatments. The recommendation supporting primary prevention sounded an older note in public health care in the midst of reports that were focused on disease containment strategies (see the following section for discussion).

B) The 1994 WHO Consultation

The first of the WHO's formal consultations in response to the 1992 IOM report occurred in April 1994–4 months after the Canada–USA meeting at Lac Tremblant. The consultation took place at WHO headquarters in Geneva, gathering together "international experts currently dealing with the concept of emerging diseases" (WHO 1994: 2).

The WHO report from the 1994 consultation noted that the USA and Canada had already begun programme development specific to EID and called for WHO's participation in these international efforts (WHO 1994: 2). The CDC document *Addressing Emerging Infectious Disease Threats* had in fact, as noted previously, called for building an international consortium tied to ministries of health, one "possibly chaired by the WHO" (CDC 1994: 21). The CDC was clearly contemplating the formation of another international health organization that would compete with WHO, or was at least threatening to do so.

WHO's international consultations on EID took place in the broader context of an international debate about how to reform WHO that was occurring in medical journals, foundations, and among its Member States

(Godlee 1994). WHO was criticized for being inefficient and having weak leadership. It was asked what role WHO should have in relation to the many new international health actors such as large private foundations? What kind of health priorities should guide international policy development after the end of the Cold War? Concerns about the ability of WHO to address EID were part of this more general debate about WHO's authority and competence, one that had the potential to lead to the marginalization of WHO within international health (Kickbusch 2000: 983).

There were 22 invited participants at the 1994 WHO consultation ("temporary advisers" in WHO parlance), 10 from the USA. Both Joshua Lederberg and Stephen Morse attended, as did Robert Shope. Lederberg served as Chair of the WHO consultation. Ruth Berkelman presented the CDC's position. Joe Losos, the sole consultant from Canada, represented the LCDC. The participants' list differed from that of the Lac Tremblant workshop as it had representation from outside Canada and the USA, notably representation from the global South such as Drs. K. Banerjee (Director, National Institute of Virology, Pune, India), N. Bhamarapravati (President Emeritus, Centre for Vaccine Development, Mahidol University, Thailand), F. Nkrumah (Director, Noguchi Memorial Institute, Accra, Ghana), and P. Tukei (Director, Virus Research Centre, Kenya Medical Research Institute, Nairobi, Kenya). WHO participants numbered 11, including James LeDuc and Giorgio Torrigiani, both of whom had attended the Lac Tremblant meeting.

The welcoming address by Ralph Henderson, Assistant Director-General of WHO, noted that WHO had a long history of dealing with new pathogens, communicable diseases, and international collaboration. Henderson stated that WHO was committed to mobilizing for the control of EID, an initiative that would be located in the Division of Communicable Diseases (WHO 1994: 13–14). A number of those who had contributed to the formation of the EID concept and national implementation strategies then held the floor. Joshua Lederberg's address attempted to bridge between the U.S. domestic audience intended by the 1992 IOM report and international public health concerns, confident of a broad overlap (WHO 1994: 3). Ruth Berkelman's comments reiterated the main points of the CDC's *Addressing Emerging Infectious Disease Threats* and emphasized the need for global cooperative action. Joe Losos summarized Canadian work on a national EID strategy. Polly Harrison (IOM) described the IOM's work since the publication of *Emerging Infections*.

The discussion that followed these presentations framed them as coming from the "developed world" and suggested that a more "global perspective" was desirable as "the same problems are being experienced in developing countries" (WHO 1994: 5), with some African nations being concerned with malaria, tuberculosis, and yellow fever. There was one suggestion to link EID with national development (WHO 1994: 5), a socio-economic strategy that had not occurred to those formulating EID in the global North, where EID had been posed primarily in relation to shoring up public health funding in national and subnational budgets.

WHO as an institution contextualized EID differently than the U.S. and Canadian presenters. The report of the 1994 ad hoc consultation contains a brief background paragraph discussing EID in relation to the history of WHO in communicable disease control, stating that this had been the focus of its work up to the 1970s but not thereafter "due to changes in health care priorities, diminished resources, and the need to focus limited manpower and fiscal resources on nontraditional communicable diseases such as HIV/AIDS" (WHO 1994: 2). The other health care priorities included the Health for All strategy that endorsed health promotion through community development. Health for All promotion was definitively sidelined in international health policy during the early to mid-1990s for a number of reasons (Kickbusch 2000: 983 and 2003a; Thomas & Weber 2004), one of which was the political challenge posed by EID. To address EID, WHO stated it would need to renew its capacity in communicable disease prevention and control (WHO 1994: 1).

The recommendations of the 1994 WHO ad hoc consultation were phrased in terms of four goals meant to revitalize WHO's communicable disease programming while emphasizing EID containment. The leading recommendation repeated the emphasis on surveillance found in the previous U.S. and Canadian reports on EID, though spatializing EID as global: "Goal 1: Strengthen Global Surveillance of Infectious Diseases" (WHO 1994: 8). The second recommendation called for enhancing the "International Infrastructure Necessary to Recognize, Report and Respond to Emerging Infectious Diseases" (WHO 1994: 10) by improving laboratory capacity, training, and communications. The third and fourth goals called for applied research and general strengthening of the global capacity for infectious disease prevention and control (WHO 1994: 11–12). In the report of the 1994 ad hoc WHO consultation, EID was first clearly put on the international health agenda. But if EID was incorporated in the second recommendation of the 1994 report to the 1994 WHO consultation, the relation between strengthening general communicable disease control and EID was not specified in the recommendations or the report as a whole. This lack of conceptual clarity in the relation between EID and communicable diseases was to characterize the subsequent history of the EID concept.

C) The 1995 WHO Consultation

The second WHO ad hoc consultation on EID took place in Geneva on January 12 and 13, 1995, 9 months after the first consultation. Of the nine international participants, only two were from the USA: Ruth Berkelman (CDC) and Stephen Morse (the Rockefeller University). Joe Losos (LCDC, Canada) chaired the meeting. Twenty-six members of the WHO secretariat attended; these included James LeDuc and Giorgio Torrigiani (who had attended the Lac Tremblant consultation and the first WHO ad hoc consultation). In his opening statement to the meeting, Ralph Henderson (WHO 1995: Appendix 1) presented the participants with one main task: how to respond to the CDC's *Addressing Emerging Infectious Disease Threats*— specifically, how to develop better international surveillance networks to deal with EID. Quoting a passage from *Addressing Emerging Infectious Disease Threats* about the organizational structure that would be needed to support international EID surveillance, Henderson directed the consultation to discuss the framework for a global consortium and an international steering committee to deal with EID. Henderson additionally requested the meeting to consider activities already begun at WHO. Having been directed to propose terms of reference for a global consortium and an international expert steering committee, the consultation did precisely this in its recommendations, which concentrated on suggestions for modifying the WHO's organizational structure in order to accommodate the recommendations of the prior ad hoc consultation in 1994.

The tone of the 1995 ad hoc meeting differed from the 1994 consultation in presenting WHO as a credible and competent actor in international public health. By way of example, the report of the 1995 consultation contained a background statement that carefully presented WHO as rising to the occasion and taking on the leadership role in EID control that had been suggested for it in the IOM's *Emerging Infections* and the CDC's *Addressing Emerging Infectious Disease Threats*. The 1995 consultation began with brief presentations about existing WHO programming in such areas as malaria control, HIV/AIDS surveillance, and zoonoses (diseases transmitted from animals to humans); this had the effect of interpreting previous WHO activities in light of the new disease category, EID, and constructing WHO as a competent actor with a long history of EID control. These presentations interpreted a number of WHO activities that had been undertaken without reference to EID as part of EID detection and control: an exercise in linguistic pragmatics.

D) A Strategic Plan

In October 1995 WHO established the Division of Emerging and other Communicable Diseases Surveillance and Control (EMC) and abolished the Division of Communicable Diseases. In order to review a 5-year strategic plan for EMC, a third WHO ad hoc consultation was convened in 1996. The overarching objective of the consultation was to provide WHO with assistance in order to "strengthen global communicable disease surveillance and control" (WHO 1996: 11). The leading recommendations of the 1994 and 1996 WHO consultations were identical: to improve global surveillance of infectious/communicable diseases and EID.

The finalized EMC strategic plan resulting from the third consultation (1996) contains a note in its last paragraph: "After the start of the programme [EMC], the group [of international experts] was enlarged at a third ad hoc meeting, organized by the Rockefeller Foundation, which reviewed this strategic plan and the EMC Summary of Programme Activities and Budget, 1996–1997" (WHO 1996: 11). We were, however, unable to locate the list of participants. Unlike the reports of 1994 and 1995, the list of participants at the third (1996) meeting is not included in the strategic plan posted on the WHO Web site, which refers readers to http://www.who.int.emc "[f]or more information".[8] This site in turn reroutes readers to the English home page of Epidemic and Pandemic Alert and Response (http://www.who.int/esr/en). There is a great deal of information about EMC on the WHO Web site, but no list of participants at the third ad hoc meeting is posted there. It might be observed that the WHO Website, like UN Web-sites overall, is so poorly organized that one can never be sure of what it does and does not contain. So too one can never prove a negative. One of our research participants recalled a meeting at the Rockefeller University in New York City (WHO Interview) related to planning for EMC, but the Rockefeller Foundation was unable to confirm the meeting, noting that records of the foundation's activities in the last 20 years are not available to the public (standard archival procedure). The Rockefeller Foundation has a long history of funding international health (W.H. Schneider 2002).

In the 1996 EMC strategic plan, WHO took the opportunity to state its strengths in communicable disease surveillance and control, listing "assets" that were diplomatic and collaborative: global information exchange, mandate from WHO Member States, WHO country representation (through offices of WHO country representatives and through WHO Regional Offices), WHO collaborating centers, and a panel of international experts (WHO 1996: 10–11). Against the temptations of incipient U.S. imperial ambition in EID control, WHO asserted its historical strengths as a UN agency for international cooperation. The EMC strategic plan represents a victory in international diplomacy for WHO, placing international EID surveillance and control under the leadership of WHO and other international public health agencies such as the Pan American Health Organization (PAHO).[9] The effect of this agreement on WHO was to renew its activities in communicable disease prevention and control, prioritizing EID.

The 1996 EMC strategic plan contained a box that defined the "EMC Vision for the 21st Century" as having one primary objective: "[a] world on alert and able to contain communicable diseases" (WHO 1996: n.p.). The "EMC Vision for the 21st Century" outlined how a world on alert was to be realized in a manner that was very close to the recommendations of the first ad hoc consultation in 1994, although it substituted "communicable disease" for "infectious diseases" and reordered the third and fourth goals. EMC's strategic goals for attaining a world on alert were: (1) "to strengthen global surveillance of communicable diseases" (WHO 1996: 3); (2) to enhance the capacity of national and international public health "infrastructure" to recognize, report, and respond to "emerging communicable diseases" (WHO 1996: 6); (3) to "strengthen national and international capacity for the prevention and control of communicable diseases" (WHO 1996: 7); and (4) to increase support for and research into communicable disease control (WHO 1996: 9). EMC's overall mission was "to strengthen national and international capacity in the surveillance and control of communicable diseases, including those that represent new, emerging and re-emerging public health problems" (WHO 1996: 3). Knowledge of communicable disease outbreaks was to be rapid and electronically mediated, making response to outbreaks possible within 24 hours of notification. The EMC mission statement presents EID as a subset of communicable diseases, although the relation between whole and part is not explicitly discussed. We will conceptualize the 'world on alert' more closely in the text to follow.

One of our research participants described the "EMC Vision for the 21st Century" as effective in orienting early work at EMC on global surveillance, outbreak response, and the IHR:

> We were always working with a vision which we developed in 1996 which was a world on alert and able to respond to communicable diseases within 24 hours using the most up-to-date communications technology, something to that effect. And that vision always stayed at the forefront as we went through the syndromic and finally fell on a new way. We found syndromic was much too sensitive to get what we needed. And so we went on to the outbreak verification through the Global Alert and Response Network. So we just did it as sort of a vision in front and working towards attaining that vision. (WHO Interview)

This research participant spoke of the EMC vision as something that oriented work, a standard that carried action forward across differing initiatives. "Syndromic" in this interview passage refers to 'syndromic surveillance,' an outbreak detection technique that tries to identify clusters that may indicate outbreak in data sources not developed for public health uses (e.g., data from stock markets, hospital emergency departments, and nonprescription sales in pharmacies). EMC planning had first identified syndromic surveillance as the route to outbreak detection, later deciding it was not effective for global surveillance (see Chapter 3 for discussion).

By 1995 mobilization around the EID concept had initiated major policy and organizational change at WHO related to communicable disease control. The formation of WHO's Division of Emerging and other Communicable Diseases Surveillance and Control in October 1995 occurred under the mandate of the World Health Assembly, the legislative body of WHO. In 1995 Resolution 48.13, *Communicable disease prevention and control: new, emerging and re-emerging infectious diseases*, was passed (World Health Assembly 1995b) with EID incorporated in the naming of the resolution. Its preamble expresses concern "at the lack of coordinated global surveillance to monitor, report and respond to *new, emerging, and re-emerging infectious diseases* [italics added]" (World Health Assembly 1995b). The first recommendation found in Resolution 48.13 was also framed in terms of EID, urging WHO country members to "strengthen national and local programmes of active surveillance for infectious diseases, ensuring that efforts are directed to early detection of outbreaks and prompt identification of *new, emerging and re-emerging infectious diseases* [italics added]" (World Health Assembly 1995b). Resolution 48.13 also requested that WHO act to "improve recognition and response to *new, emerging, and re-emerging infectious diseases* [italics added] in a manner sustainable by all countries" (World Health Assembly 1995b). The year 1995 also marked the important World Health Assembly resolution calling for the revision of the IHR (1969). Resolution WHA48.7, *Revision and Updating of the International Health Regulations* (World Health Assembly 1995a), identifies itself as "WHO's initiative on *new, emerging and re-emerging infectious diseases* [italics added]" (World Health Assembly 1995a). The revision of the IHR (1969) in WHA48.7 is motivated in the same terms as the same genetic and ecological reasoning that had characterized the EID conception in the 1992 IOM report, naming the following as causes pertinent to the call for revising the IHR (1969): "continuous evolution in the public health threat posed by infectious diseases related to the agents themselves, to their easier transmission in changing physical and social environments, and to diagnostic and treatment capacities" (World Health Assembly 1995a). This resolution also called attention to the fact that the IHR (1969) applied to only three diseases (plague, cholera, and yellow fever) after smallpox was declared eradicated in 1980.

The stabilities of the older framework covering "pestilential diseases" that had dominated international public health law since the end of the 19th century made little sense to planning for EID, which was concerned with potentiality and the emergent in communicable diseases. The 1996 EMC report to the World Health Assembly on the IHR noted a conflict between EID control and the IHR (1969):

> [T]hey [the IHR] fail to regulate procedures necessary for the management of new and re-emerging diseases, especially those which are an international threat. Global coordination is still vitally needed for such purposes as monitoring, reporting, and response. The experts considered that the international control of infectious diseases is more effective if undertaken through improved surveillance and intervention strategies than if quarantine measures are applied at sites distant from the source of infection.[10]

Calls from within and without the WHO system to revise the IHR (1969) have a history that dates to the point of their adoption (Dorolle 1968; Roelsgaard 1974; Velimirovic 1976; see Chapter 4 for discussion). The many critiques of the redundancy of the IHR (1969) and of poor compliance with their terms by Member States repeatedly failed to generate the required momentum to lead to any real change in international health law. Only with the reimagining of infectious disease through the EID concept (and the later impetus of the global SARS outbreak in 2002) were discursive conditions set that could mobilize an international commitment to remake the Regulations.

EID formed the conceptual impetus to the formation of a global emergency vigilance apparatus. The expansiveness of EID and the sense of urgency it provoked refashioned international infectious disease control. The remarkable organizing force behind the politically backed EID concept is demonstrated by the speed with which it was taken up within national and international public health circles. As we have shown, by 1995 the EID concept was effecting organizational change at WHO, linked to the programmatic vision of a world on alert. This is remarkable given that "emerging infectious diseases" had made its first appearance in WHO's *Weekly Epidemiological Record* only during 1993 in reports based on articles from the CDC's *Morbidity and Mortality Weekly Report* ("Emerging Infectious Diseases" 1993a, 1993b). By 1996 the EID concept had been so thoroughly internationalized for the purposes of medical research that in January of that year, 36 medical journals in 21 nation-states did a special issue on the theme of emerging and reemerging infectious disease. Nicholas King (2001: 2) termed this "the first global theme issue," one that was "unprecedented in the history [of] medical publishing." The 1992 IOM report *Emerging Infections* had a wild success with the EID concept, its hyperbole having motivated institutional change in communicable disease control nationally and internationally. Just 3 years had passed from the invention of the EID concept to the transformation of communicable disease policy and organization at WHO.

E) A Vigilance Apparatus

The notion of a "world on alert" that was expressed in the "EMC Vision for the 21st Century" proposed a new approach for dealing with international infectious disease outbreaks, the first comprehensive policy statement for what we conceptualize as a global emergency vigilance apparatus. Here we seek a closer conceptualization of the initial discursive characteristics of the world on alert: its target, temporal modality, goal, and relation to the category of communicable disease.

The world on alert is a vigilance apparatus on constant watch worldwide to detect outbreaks, issue alerts, and respond on a 24-hour basis to prevent international epidemics. Communicable disease outbreaks form the target of the world on alert in the EMC mission statement. The temporal modality of WHO's outbreak knowledge is made synchronous with outbreak in order to make possible a 24-hour response time after detection.

This temporal modality was later routinely called "real time" or "near real time" in public health (see Chapter 5 for discussion).

The relation in the 1996 strategic plan between communicable disease and EID is whole to part, as one can see in EMC's name: Emerging and other Communicable Diseases Surveillance and Control. Given the conventions of written English, it would appear that EID is more significant than other communicable diseases. With this division in the communicable disease concept between emerging and other, EMC is given the mandate to know about and respond to not just a fixed set of known diseases, but also to new and emerging communicable diseases. In the world on alert, WHO's communicable disease programming acquired responsibility for microbial diseases in their virtuality/potentiality.

National and international public health systems in a world on alert have a global capacity to "contain communicable diseases" (WHO 1996: n.p.). To accomplish this goal, the world on alert requires the creation of a new technical apparatus. The EMC vision statement emphasized the need for strong national surveillance systems, global monitoring networks, rapid electronic information exchange, and national and international preparedness and response to "contain epidemics of international importance." From the 1992 IOM report onwards the EID concept was associated with calls for a detection technique that could quickly and continuously monitor for outbreaks at a global level in order to contain them.

The world on alert has the capacity to identify and contain infectious disease outbreaks prior to their international transmission. Alertness is oriented to the overarching goal of containment, which (see Chapter 1) has a technical meaning in public health: maintaining "regional eradication of infectious disease" by preventing transmission of a disease from areas in which it is endemic to an area in which it has been eradicated (Last 2001: 39). Public health personnel also speak of containing a particular epidemic/outbreak in the sense of preventing its transmission beyond a designated area, for instance, one that has been quarantined. Global-level infectious disease containment in either sense requires the international coordination of public health efforts. The overriding goal of the world on alert—to contain communicable diseases—falls on a North–South cleavage in terms of world power as the chief areas of endemic communicable diseases to be contained are found in the global South. Containment thus has a geopolitical spatial organization. Yet the goal of containment is simultaneously a cosmopolitan and humanitarian one of reducing sickness and death from acute and infectious diseases worldwide.

The relation of emergency response and assistance—tactics of disease containment in a world on alert—to communicable disease prevention is an ongoing problem in international public health that has a long history of internal debate at WHO.[11] In our interview research, WHO participants reported that they experienced conflict in the field between their organizational mandate for disease containment and their duty as physicians to treat patients. One research participant posed this position as a tension between disease containment and humanitarianism:

> We are responsible through the IHR for maintaining international health security in the area of epidemics. But WHO has a primary mandate also, and that is a humanitarian mandate to reduce the suffering of people from all diseases, including infectious diseases. So when we go to the field to deal with an Ebola outbreak we have to deal with what are essentially two demands on the organization. In my view, the primary demand is to aid the suffering people who are dying from the epidemic diseases, and the other demand is the demand of the international community that that disease be contained. And that sometimes is very difficult to manage actually. (WHO Interview)

The goal of disease containment may sometimes be in tension with patient care:

> Containment and care don't always completely match each other. Containing people with Ebola may mean just putting them into a room and letting them die. You've contained the outbreak. You've stopped it being an international threat, but you have done nothing to reduce the suffering of those individuals or their family . . . And I do think we've become more sophisticated at balancing our needs to be humanitarians and to assist the government at easing the suffering of their people and at the same time fulfilling an international mandate to contain the disease. But it's a duality we live in and you can't get around it. (WHO Interview)

Our research participants gave witness to the ethically difficult positions in which some of them had been placed as physicians when containing outbreak.[12]

Containment, the goal of the world on alert, is supported by North and South, though for differing reasons according to our WHO research participants:

LW/EM: "Emerging infectious diseases" came out of the United States and it was originally very tied to American national interests. How did the concept shift at the WHO?

WHO Research Participant: Well, it shifted because the Director-General saw the importance of . . . an emerging diseases program, and then the program was able to sell it as a public health security issue to other industrialized countries. It's never been a big concern for developing countries. . . . If you can get the politicians to focus on public health security, that infectious diseases are a security issue—and we spent a lot of time on that, a lot of writing on that—you soon end up with a broader agenda than just the U.S. agenda.

LW/EM: And so that would shift the perception of emerging diseases as a First World concern?

WHO *Research Participant:* No. I think it's always been a First World concern. And it still is. In the North, it's a concern for security; you don't want those diseases to come in and harm their economies and their people. In developing countries it's an issue of prevent our people from dying and prevent the economic repercussions that occur when they do start. So the win–win is detect and respond to infectious diseases where they're occurring—and that's a win for everybody. (WHO Interview)

This research participant frames EID as primarily a global North concern related to disease transmission from the South that could damage health security in the North. For those in the global South, EID is perceived as occurring inside their national territorial borders, with a consequent need to prevent economic sanctions from outside and to "prevent our people from dying." Detection and response at the source is represented as the solution to these heterogeneous interpretations of emerging diseases, bridging differing positions in a world order viewed from the perspective of the world on alert.

Another research participant forcefully pointed to differences in North–South perspectives on infectious disease outbreaks:

I think the brutal reality is that the North cares about the South and the area of epidemic diseases primarily because of security and not necessarily because of humanitarianism. . . . People think the people of the South are only interested in the humanitarian aspects of how an epidemic affects their population. . . . It's not true now because many of the economies in the South and Africa and Asia are selling products and moving people into the North . . . if they're seen to export disease, that is a very negative thing not only in terms of development in their own country but in terms of their economic security. (WHO Interview)

This participant sees the North as orienting to epidemic disease in terms of "security," while the South is concerned about the perception that it might be exporting epidemic disease for fear of the impact this might have on development and economic stability.

We have analyzed the world on alert as the first formulation of global emergency vigilance. Later work in the period between 2002 and 2005 built on the discursive characteristics of the world on alert, including its real-time temporal modality, conceptualization of communicable diseases as both actual and potential/virtual, and a double and contradictory goal of

containment that serves the regional interests of the North while simultaneously being oriented to reducing the burden of infectious diseases for all the
peoples of the world. Later work also the established target of global health
surveillance—disease outbreak. As articulated by the strategic vision for
EMC, the world on alert targets communicable disease outbreaks, not the
later target of "public health emergencies of international concern." The
concept of public health emergencies of international concern appears in
the IHR (2005), but had been introduced into WHO work at least as early
as 2002 (see Chapter 4, p. 122–123 for discussion). International public
health emergencies as defined in the IHR (2005) include chemical, environmental, industrial, and radiological disasters; outbreaks of foodborne disease; and the public health impact of bioweapons use (WHO 2007: 17–33).
The EMC vision of a world on alert opened up a process of dramatically
expanding the target of international infectious disease control. However,
in its formal expression by the EMC, the target of a world on alert was
limited to communicable diseases, not emergencies. Unlike the later emergency vigilance apparatus, the world on alert did not, at the outset, include
bioweapons as part of its target, nor was it securitized.[13]

The Power/Knowledge Relations of EID

To link the EID concept with anything other than the compassionate alleviation of suffering provokes surprise and resistance. Who would not support action against EID? Such has been the success of the EID concept and
associated health policy that it has become a self-evident good. Yet public
health is a field that generates competing conceptual and policy alternatives
for securing collective health. The primary objective of global emergency
vigilance—containment—stands in tension with alternative approaches
that seek to promote health through primary health care or a social determinants of health approach.

We close this chapter by calling attention to two power/knowledge
effects associated with the EID concept that fall on the North–South
division. First, we argue that EID is conceptually unstable in relation to
the wider concept of communicable disease, an instability that reflects
North–South differences in public health. Second, increased spending on
development assistance for health since the mid-1990s has targeted EID,
a practice of vertical (disease-specific) development assistance that has
been questioned as creating problems for national health system planning
in the South.

A) Conceptual Instability

The EID concept is a distinction introduced into a prior field of public
health concepts. It is an unstable concept that is used in contradictory

senses and also has an unsettled and uncertain relation to the concept of communicable disease.

The relation of the EID concept to the concept of communicable/infectious disease is not dealt with explicitly in the 1992 IOM report, making the relation between the two terms uncertain. The IOM's *Emerging Infections* does refer to infectious diseases throughout, implicitly treating EID as having greater domestic public health significance than other infectious diseases. A rigorous application of the IOM's (1992) definition of EID as a rise in the incidence of an infectious disease has the effect of dividing the prior notion of communicable diseases into two notions: the new, emerging, and re-emerging diseases versus those communicable diseases that are not new, emerging, and re-emerging (i.e., those communicable diseases that have a constant or declining incidence). Logically speaking, endemic diseases whose incidence rates are not increasing are not EID. Where an infectious disease has a high and constant incidence or prevalence, a condition called 'hyperendemic,' it would not then be an EID—and by implication, it would not be of concern to the public health policy of the USA and its allies.

As we mentioned in the introduction to this chapter, Paul Farmer (1999), a physician with a long history of treating tuberculosis in Haiti (where tuberculosis is hyperendemic) has been strongly critical of the EID concept, arguing that it is inappropriate to the understanding of infectious disease in the global South. However, because tuberculosis is increasing in incidence globally and multidrug resistant variants are also on the rise, tuberculosis anywhere in the world is often considered an EID. Arguments from the global burden of disease have resulted in the classification of HIV/AIDS, tuberculosis, and malaria as EIDs (IOM 2003: 25–32). The EID concept is a plastic one that sometimes results in the suspension of universalist epidemiological criteria in order to accommodate arguments from absolute numbers.

EID thus has two contradictory aspects: (1) as a perspectival concept sensitive to variation in local, regional, and national disease incidence; and (2) as a globally invariant list of infectious diseases. These might respectively be termed the 'relative' and 'absolute' variants of the EID concept. There is an additional and separate question of global justice in relation to the application of the EID concept. On the one hand, global public health necessitates finding some means by which to distinguish infectious diseases that cross national boundaries and that pose international health threats from those diseases that do not have these characteristics. On the other hand, once those internationally significant infectious diseases are identified, their priority can be questioned in terms of high mortality from hyperendemic (and holoendemic[14]) diseases amongst the poorest countries on earth. This question, a political one of global justice, may not be fully resolvable at the present time, but we argue that the EID concept assists in obfuscating it.

The conceptual relation between EID and other communicable diseases shifts across national and international reports. In the important WHO report that lays out a biregional communicable disease control strategy for the Western Pacific and South-East Asia, *Asia Pacific Strategy for Emerging Diseases*, EID is defined in the Terminology section as including "the so-called new diseases, as well as the re-emerging and resurging known diseases, and *known epidemic-prone diseases* [italics added]" (WHO 2005: 15). The first sentence of this report asserts that "[i]n Asia and the Pacific, emerging diseases *and other epidemic-prone diseases* [italics added] pose serious public health threats to many Member States" (WHO 2005: 2). The inclusion of "other epidemic-prone diseases" in the definition of EID reconstructs its meaning, adapting the EID concept for use in the Western Pacific and South-East Asia: an exercise in the recontextualization of EID for the South.

Examples of conceptual instability in the relation of EID to other communicable diseases occur in the CDC journal *Emerging Infectious Diseases*, which publishes country-specific profiles of EID. Authors writing profiles of local or national regions in the South either do not use the EID concept or contextualize EID in relation to regional communicable/infectious diseases. In the article "Emerging Infectious Diseases in Mongolia" (Ebright, Altantsetseg, & Oyungerel 2003), the EID concept that appears in the title does not appear in the text of the article. The authors instead use the concept of infectious diseases, summarizing basic public health data on mortality from the main infectious diseases in Mongolia, and describing the main public health measures used to control these diseases. A similar though more complex pattern is found in a second article, "Emerging Infectious Diseases—Southeast Asia" (Lam 1998) by Dr. Sai Kit Lam, head of the Department of Medical Microbiology, Faculty of Medicine, at the University of Malay (Kuala Lumpur, Malaysia). This article uses the concept of infectious disease rather than EID, although the author does refer to disease emergence, emerging diseases, and new infectious diseases. Although entitled "Emerging Infectious Diseases—Southeast Asia," Lam's article is not organized around the EID concept, nor does the text sharply distinguish between infectious diseases and EID. Thus, by way of example, after Lam summarizes global statistics on deaths in 1995 from respiratory diseases (including pneumonia), diarrhoeal diseases (including cholera, typhoid, and dysentery), tuberculosis, malaria, hepatitis B, and measles, he observes that "[f]aced with the reality of infectious diseases on a daily basis, Southeast Asia nations have not been able to give emerging diseases surveillance the priority it deserves" (Lam 1998: 145) and follows with a discussion of infectious diseases such as polio, aseptic meningitis, and dengue fever. A discrepancy between title and text is found in both these articles, which are briefing papers on mortality from communicable diseases in world regions having high levels of endemic communicable diseases.

The relation between the EID concept and the communicable disease concept is also unstable in terms of part/whole relations. EID may be conceptualized as a subset of communicable diseases, as did Ralph Henderson in his opening remarks to the 1994 WHO ad hoc consultation, where he clarified the relation between EID and communicable diseases by noting that "most diseases currently being discussed as 'emerging' fall under the broad category of communicable diseases" (WHO 1994: 14). While Canadian and U.S. representatives to the 1994 WHO consultation spoke in terms of "new, emerging and re-emerging infectious diseases," WHO included EIDs within communicable diseases, inventing the phrase "emerging communicable diseases." WHO itself has a general pattern of opting for 'communicable disease' in preference to 'EID.' Thus, by way of example, the carefully named Division of Emerging and other Communicable Diseases Surveillance and Control was renamed Communicable Diseases in 1998. As part of a general reorganization of WHO headquarters structure, Communicable Diseases was in turn renamed Health Security and Environment in 2008, a displacement of the communicable disease concept by a security concept.

EID is sometimes equated with all communicable diseases, thus displacing and substituting for the category of communicable diseases. We have seen examples of the displacement of the communicable disease concept and its substitution by EID immediately above in the CDC journal *Emerging Infectious Diseases*. The substitution of the EID concept for the concept of communicable diseases is an interpretive move that constitutes the historical experience and periodization of communicable diseases in the global North as globally normative. This strips the EID concept of perspective and context, removing the burden of explaining emerging diseases in relation to other communicable diseases.

Marilyn Strathern (1995) observes that the global forms its own context in part by rendering obscure its own political, economic, cultural, and social conditions. She additionally argues that the global is produced through new universal constructions that enable specific forms of connection. Her argument is illustrated by the movement of the EID concept from its formation and meaning in a U.S. national context to its recontexualization in global health where it signifies a universal connectedness postulated through vulnerability to EID. The global is as well a space of interpretative contestations formed in reaction to the dominance of perspectives that conceive of themselves as relationless and contextless: universal. Thus, under conditions wherein the meaning of EID is equated with all communicable diseases, public health officials in the global South react to and revise the EID concept, a struggle over the institutional control of meaning that recontextualizes EID in relation to other communicable diseases. Struggles over conceptualizing the meaning of EID in relation to other infectious/communicable diseases reflect North–South differences in collective health within the global political and economic order.

B) EID and Development Assistance for Health

International development assistance for health in the late 1990s and early 2000s was characterized by a pattern of prioritizing funding for a small number of high-profile EIDs. A comprehensive WHO collaborative study begins by stating unequivocally that "[s]ince 2000, the emergence of several large disease-specific global health initiatives (GHIs) has changed the way in which international donors provide assistance for health" (World Health Organization Maximizing Positive Synergies Collaborative Group 2009). How such disease-specific or 'vertical' funding affects the general health systems of beneficiary countries has since become the subject of international debate, although concerns about the impact of disease-specific programming, now often called 'global health initiatives,' long predate the invention of the EID concept. In an important statement, Halfdan Mahler, Director-General of WHO from 1973 to 1988, drew on his experiences of having helped to establish a national tuberculosis programme in India in order to describe a number of problems associated with disease-specific initiatives. These included human resource problems related to the shortage of trained health workers and related challenges associated with integrating a vertical TB programme with general health services (Uplekar & Raviglione 2007; Mahler 1966).

Criticisms and debates about vertical programmes have been reinvigorated of late, partly in response to the emergence of new international donors that fund disease-specific programmes in the global South, particularly those directed toward HIV/AIDS. New funders since 1999 include the Global Fund to Fight AIDS, Tuberculosis and Malaria (Global Fund), the Global Alliance for Vaccines and Immunization (GAVI Alliance), the World Bank MAP (Multi-Country HIV/AIDS Program for Africa), and the U.S. President's Emergency Plan for AIDS Relief (PEPFAR). These are the four largest donors of international development assistance for disease-specific work. The Global Fund was formed in 2001 as a public-private partnership to provide funding, as its title would indicate, in the area of HIV/AIDS, tuberculosis, and malaria. The GAVI Alliance was founded as a public-private partnership in 2000 to provide access to immunization in poor countries. Established in 2003, PEPFAR describes itself as "the largest commitment by any nation to combat a single disease in human history" (United States President's Emergency Plan for AIDS Relief 2009).[15] Begun in 1999, the World Bank MAP programme is a response to HIV/AIDS in sub-Saharan Africa. These four organizations are thus all involved with development assistance for EID—the Global Fund, PEPFAR, and the World Bank MAP exclusively so—with the GAVI Alliance funding both EID and communicable disease immunization more broadly. To give some idea of scale, we note that in 2007 the Global Fund and GAVI contributed US$2.16 billion in international development funding for disease-specific initiatives and PEPFAR US$5.4 billion (World Health Organization Maximizing Positive Synergies Collaborative Group 2009). World Bank MAP expended a total of US $1.8 billion on HIV/AIDS programming from 1999 to June 2009.[16]

It is commonplace to say that spending on international assistance for health, particularly in the area of infectious disease control, has increased since the late 1990s, but it is harder to get reliable numbers. A careful study of the impact of global health initiatives on recipient national health care systems published in *The Lancet* (World Health Organization Maximizing Positive Synergies Collaborative Group 2009) states that between 2001 and 2006, official development assistance for health increased from US$5.6 billion to US$18.8 billion per year, with additional funding from private sources such as the Bill and Melinda Gates Foundation. The Organisation for Economic Co-operation and Development (OECD) estimates that during 2005 to 2006 HIV/AIDS control comprised 35% of total multilateral and bilateral aid to health; TB, malaria, and other infectious disease control comprised an additional 16% of total aid in that year (OECD-DAC 2008: Chart 3, "Sub-Sectoral Breakdown of Aid to Health").[17] Combined, these OECD figures indicate that 51% of official development assistance for health was allocated to infectious disease control in the period between 2005 and 2006, most of it in the area of what is considered EID (HIV/AIDS, tuberculosis, and malaria). In the period from FY2004 to FY2008, U.S. development assistance commitments in the USAID Global Health Programmes allocated 21% of funding for infectious diseases to child health and survival, maternal health, and family planning (US$4.6 billion) and 79% to HIV, TB, and malaria (US$17.7 billion), which again illustrates the allocation of funds to EID over other communicable diseases.[18]

A critique of the activities of global health initiatives is now well established, having recently appeared in the pages of *Foreign Affairs*, the *British Medical Journal*, and the *Financial Times* (Garrett 2007; England 2007, 2008; Jack 2007). Critics have argued that current international disease-specific funding emphasizes a narrow range of diseases at the expense of competing local health priorities. Concerns have been raised about the flow of health care personnel and resources from general primary health services to internationally funded disease-specific programmes, leading to poorly integrated and coordinated health services and planning in beneficiary countries. Others have argued that the multiplicity of donors has created a situation of poor global coordination in international health, an excessively complex global funding architecture with conflicting reporting and accountability requirements, and a lack of national control over planning health systems in the global South (Stilberschmidt, Matheson, & Kickbusch 2008; Schieber, Fleisher, & Gottret 2006). These and related concerns about the impact of international vertical health funding are currently under discussion at the International Health Partnership, a coordinating body for development assistance in health that consists of eight private and public international health agencies: WHO; World Bank; the GAVI Alliance; UNICEF; UNFPA; the Global Fund to Fight AIDS, Tuberculosis and Malaria; and the Bill and Melinda Gates Foundation.[19] Concerns have also been brought forward as a part of calls to transform the architecture of global health funding in the direction of 'diagonal' financing that emphasizes the potential for vertical funding to generate disease-specific as well as 'spill over' or generalized health system improvements (Ooms, Van Damme, Baker, Zeitz, & Schrecker 2008; Frenk 2008).

The call for 'diagonal thinking' to resolve the sharp polarization of the debate about the relationship between HIV/AIDS-specific funding and global health systems strengthening was a prominent feature of the 2008 International AIDS Conference (hereinafter AIDS 2008). Conference organizers strategically featured a number of special sessions addressing the critique of HIV/AIDS-specific global health initiatives, largely in response to the criticisms made by Laurie Garrett and Roger England of global HIV/AIDS funding.[20] A year prior to the conference Garrett had argued that HIV/AIDS-specific international health aid had created "cadres of healthcare workers who function largely independently from countries' other health-related systems" (2007: 14–17). Roger England went so far as to call for immediately disbanding UNAIDS and argued that global HIV/AIDS funding is excessive, ineffective and "distorts countries' efforts to deal with their problems" (2007: 565). AIDS 2008 created opportunities for replying to such criticisms and helped shift the contours of debate about contemporary disease-specific international health assistance. Michael Kazatchkine (Executive Director of the Global Fund), Mark Dybul (U.S. Global AIDS Coordinator charged with overseeing the implementation of PEPFAR), and others argued the case that HIV/AIDS-specific global health initiatives have general effects on health systems. An emphasis was placed on how vertical funding has improved population health in beneficiary countries as measured by general life expectancy and infant mortality rates, how it has also helped build an infrastructure for the delivery of primary health care, how it has helped to support and train health care personnel, to develop laboratory and procurement services, and to free up workforce time in hospitals (Kazatchkine 2008; Dybul 2008). For others, the conference was an opportunity to reinforce arguments for global health initiatives to deepen their investment in health workforce training, support, and task shifting and to emphasize enduring problems with the harmonization of independent funding streams at country level (Russel 2008; Koenders 2008). An emerging policy and research direction surfaced at AIDS 2008 that called for an end to an oversimplified bifurcation of HIV/AIDS-specific and general health services and also called for new diagonal research aimed at enhancing the integration of HIV/AIDS with tuberculosis care, sexual health services, primary health care, child and maternal care, and other foci of health services delivery.

We emphasize that our intent is not to contribute to the debate about international health assistance. At the time of writing in June 2009, the International Health Partnership is in the early stage of implementing a new development assistance model for health that has been designed to address many of the concerns we have mentioned here, including coordinating aid with national health care planning, predictable financing, and harmonization of aid across agencies. The International Health Partnership proposes to negotiate with sovereign states around agreements called "country compacts" that integrate infectious diseases prevention and control into much broader health and national macroeconomic planning (International Health Partnership 2008). Social scientists might be curious about the place of public health in a new model of international health development with a vastly expanded concept of health.

Rather that attempting a critique of development assistance for health, we aim to call attention to how much vertical development funding has been EID focused. The extent of the organization of development assistance for health around EID represents an important migration of this concept from international concerns about outbreak detection and containment to a global discursive context emphasizing health-related international development. The focus of international health development practice around EID provides further evidence of the success of EID as an active concept. But it also points to enduring conflicts internal to the EID concept at the level of its alignment with the health needs and priorities of the global South.

We have argued that the EID concept has an uncertain and indeed incoherent relation to the concept of communicable disease. Given that lists of emerging diseases will vary according to incidence in differing populations, no standard global list of EID is possible. In practice, EID refers to diseases that may be transmitted internationally and are or might become of international public health concern (see Chapter 4) as distinguished from epidemic-prone and endemic communicable diseases, primarily those of the global South. EID was not designed to conceptualize the historical experience and contemporary needs of the global South in communicable disease prevention and control. Its internal historical horizon assumes emergence from nonexistence and emergence after subsidence, rather than emergence from enduringly high levels of endemic and epidemic-prone communicable diseases. Under the former conditions, which postulate 'the health/epidemiologic transition', EID contrasts with historically low levels of communicable disease; but under the latter conditions, the normative claim that emerging diseases should have priority status in communicable disease control over endemic and epidemic-prone disease must be argued rather than treated as intuitively obvious. However, the success of the EID concept has been precisely to imagine differing regions of the world as mirroring the global North.

Conclusion

In this chapter, we have provided an account that displays EID as an active concept. The threat of EID was devised in the USA to revitalize an underfunded and politically marginalized public health system. Our discussion gives evidence of how EID was recontextualized as it moved from its site of formation in the USA to its internationalization at WHO. This process of internationalization involved a shift in the meaning of EID, as it was no longer focused on infectious disease control in the USA. It was also a process of activation of the concept with important effects at the level of WHO's engagement with an initiative that would insert a new governance apparatus into international infectious disease control. With its powerful institutional allies, the EID concept constituted an epistemological break in international communicable disease control from one oriented to known diseases to one responsible for a microbial world full of potential and surprise. Not only was the microbial world full of the actual, the emerging, and the potential, but this microbial multiplicity also had to be made governable.

From its earliest days, the EID concept took programmatic form in demands for surveillance, preparedness, collaboration, and response that operated faster and with more complete information than anything previously imagined. The EID concept was the main impetus to the formation of this world on alert, which we have treated as the first formulation of global emergency vigilance. But WHO itself has maintained a distance from the EID concept at key points, treating EID as part of communicable disease in naming the Division of Emerging and other Communicable Diseases Surveillance and Response (1995), reasserting the concept of communicable disease when this division was renamed Communicable Diseases (1998), and using "public health emergencies of international concern" in preference to EID in the IHR (2005).

The 'world on alert' represents a particular policy approach to communicable disease control. It is not a vision of prevention, and it is very far from integrating health into development. Ameliorating poverty, improving housing and employment opportunities, and decreasing the rates of chronic illnesses and injuries are types of public health programming that do not conform to a model of emergency vigilance, although they are less heroic. The triumph of the EID concept lay in presenting international communicable disease control as having stakes so manifestly imperative that they appeared above any political process. The political question with respect to global emergency vigilance is what its place should be in communicable disease budgets and in broader public health thinking and action.

3 Early Warning Outbreak Detection and Alert
A Technique

The consolidation of EID as a problem within global public health circles posed a challenge to the routine form and operation of international infectious disease control. The many reports about EID analyzed in the previous chapter (Lac Tremblant Declaration Declaration 1994; WHO 1994, 1995, 1996) all had a leading recommendation for enhanced global surveillance of infectious diseases. *Emerging Infections* (IOM 1992) and the CDC's *Addressing Emerging Infectious Disease Threats* (CDC 1994) sharply criticized WHO's leadership in the area and pressured WHO to establish EID as an organizational priority in efforts to improve global health surveillance. These reports and later WHO consultations on EID were noteworthy for the epistemological conservatism of their vision for enhanced global infectious disease control. The suggestions for responding to the new terrain of uncertain health risks problematized by the EID concept rarely strayed from the authority of the epidemiological case report. That is, they privileged communications of disease diagnoses or of agents (e.g., toxins) causing disease that were made to public health authorities in voluntary or mandatory conformity with the requirements of official reporting systems. For the most part, reports from the consultations expressed generic calls for enhanced training and expansion of existing international networks of epidemiological communication and diagnostic/laboratory capacities.

While it was clear in the early 1990s that EID meant that international detection of and response to infectious disease outbreaks needed to become much faster and that more outbreaks needed reporting, the means for realizing such changes had not yet been imagined. How were existent approaches for identifying and responding to outbreaks of infectious diseases to be transformed into a vigilance apparatus compatible with the temporal demands and response capabilities of a 'world on alert'? Vigilance depends on detection technologies that continuously gather data about highly dangerous events (such as possible meltdowns in nuclear power reactors), facilitates the review of such data by experts, and makes judgments about issuing alerts. How could international public health communication about infectious disease outbreaks be instrumentalized to accommodate the demands of an emergency vigilance apparatus?

The surprising solution developed by public health officials was to establish online news and other unofficial forms of information as the discursive foundation of a new technique for addressing international public health threats: early warning outbreak detection, alert and response. Early warning outbreak detection, alert and response is comprised of four related processes: identifying, verifying, and issuing alerts about public health events that may indicate the presence of international public health emergencies and responding to those events deemed to be so (Heymann, Rodier, & WHO Operational Support Team to the Global Outbreak Alert and Response Network 2001). In this chapter we focus on the first three processes, or what is called early warning detection and alert. Public health has long used news as a medium to exchange information about infectious disease. But early warning outbreak detection and alert enhances the organizational presence of news in international infectious disease control and, as it was later called, 'global public health security.' Early warning outbreak detection and alert responds to the demand for faster, more comprehensive outbreak and emergency information by turning to virtual sources of near 'real-time' news information that are not politically authorized by the sovereign members of WHO. In doing so it reorganizes the social relations of knowledge in international infectious disease control, standardizing and interiorizing within its apparatus news sources that were previously only sporadically used by international public health officials.

The focus of this chapter—the institutional significance of news within international infectious disease control—represents an important analytic shift for social science research on news and infectious diseases. Most social science analyses of the media and infectious diseases examine issues of representation. A common form of analysis explores the content and narrative form of news to argue that sensationalist reporting contributes to public confusion and fear about infection, obscures the role that social and economic conditions play in facilitating epidemics, stigmatizes social groups associated with infectious diseases, and furthers morally simplistic distinctions between guilty 'carriers' and innocent 'victims' (Weldon 2001; Stabile 1997; Lupton 1994; Watney 1997). When social scientists have examined the significance of health news for broad forms of social organization, they have generally emphasized relations between modernity, reflexivity, and self-fashioning, and explored how mass-mediated images, including those communicated via the Internet, shape understandings of health and illness, act as discursive resources for identity formation, and help shift power relationships between medical experts and patients (Seale 2002, 2003; Petersen 2002; Hardey 2001)

This chapter departs from these familiar analyses by exploring the changing role news has played in the social organization of international infectious disease control. We rewrite the institutional significance of news for global infectious disease surveillance and public health security, leaving aside the argument of news as misinformation to investigate how news enters into and shapes knowledge of outbreak and other public health threats within the formal apparatus of international public health security and infectious disease control . Our analysis treats news as consequential for the way international systems that detect and respond to public health events are organized. To fashion that analysis we pay careful attention to the discursive form of news and, in particular, to developments provoked by its status as unofficial knowledge.

Organized comparatively, this chapter examines the organizational presence of news in public health knowledge of outbreak in two periods: the postcolonial period from 1946 (the formation of WHO) to 1986 (the 20-year cutoff for our archival research) and the first decade of the global emergency vigilance apparatus, which began in the late 1990s. We commence with an historical investigation of the place of news in postcolonial international outbreak communications at WHO. News, we argue, was far more important for WHO and international infectious disease control in the second half of the 20th century than has been recognized. We also emphasize that the relationship between unofficial and official forms of knowledge in public health practice in this period was complex and contested; it included both challenges to official knowledge by news media as well as the instrumental use of news reports in the everyday activities of public health authorities. We then turn to examine news in early warning outbreak detection, emphasizing how online news was incorporated into the outbreak identification activities of the Global Public Health Intelligence Network (GPHIN) and prompted the establishment of formalized verification activities at WHO in order to align alerts based on news reports with diplomatically confirmed truth. We argue that public health officials turned to establish online news as a legitimate source of outbreak information in response to the demand for timeliness posed by EID and the shaming effect of news reports that outpaced official country notification of outbreak. We end with a comparative analysis of the relation between official and unofficial sources of outbreak information in the two periods. Global public health emergency vigilance is characterized by the transformation of unofficial information of public health events into a fully actionable, parallel form of knowledge to official reporting.

Postcolonial Knowledge of Outbreak

Early warning outbreak detection can be understood as an historical break in the ways infectious disease outbreaks came into public health knowledge at WHO during the second half of the 20th century. To understand the nature of that break, one must give an historical context and thickness to public health knowledge of outbreak during the second half of the 20th century. We have been struck by how the published articles of international public health officials (Heymann 2006; Grein et al. 2000; Heymann et al. 2001; Formenty et al. 2006) and respected secondary commentators (Fidler 2004a) draw sharp contrasts between current outbreak detection and past epidemiological communications, where WHO officials had access only to epidemiological information that was often months, even years, out of date. Over the course of our research, our research participants often remarked that public health personnel formerly had access only to formal reports of outbreak officially filed by sovereign states. Unofficial information about outbreak derived from news and other sources has thus largely been considered absent from earlier forms of international communicable disease surveillance. While our own analysis emphasizes a marked shift from the late 1990s in the organizational presence of news in international infectious disease control, we are also wary of distinctions that render news vitally present now and wholly absent from earlier WHO approaches to identifying outbreak and epidemic.

Before sketching the relations between official and unofficial knowledge of outbreak at WHO prior to the late 1990s, it is necessary to know something about the historical context in which the sharp distinction was fashioned between official and unofficial, formal and informal. WHO and other agencies in the UN system were formed in the late 1940s at an historical moment of decolonization. Strong national control of epidemiological information was asserted in the postcolonial period, in contrast to the weak control that Euro-American colonies had been able to maintain over the international transmission of epidemiological information concerning infectious disease outbreaks in their territories.

Colonies did not control the epidemiological information that was broadcast about them. Of the colonial epidemiological intelligence systems, the Far Eastern Bureau (established in 1925) of the League of Nations Health Organization is the best documented, with leading work done by the historian Lenore Manderson (1995). Manderson has established that in 1931, the weekly wireless reports of the Far Eastern Bureau were broadcasting information from "56 health administrations and 156 ports" in the Western Pacific, Asia, and the Middle East (1995: 123).[1] She documented general compliance with the colonial extraction and circulation of epidemic intelligence, although she also noted a number of exceptions such as a civil war in mainland China that interrupted communications and anticolonial sentiment in Hong Kong (Manderson 1995: 123–125).[2] Wireless reports were broadcast in a telegraphic code (Brooke 1926) that applied over all areas of the Far Eastern Bureau, setting a standard of report for the colonial world. Forty-six different infectious diseases were included in this telegraphic code (Brooke 1926: 29).

Epidemiological communications at WHO broke with the older colonial organization of what was called 'epidemiological intelligence,' subjecting it to authorization by sovereign states; for this reason we have characterized the period from the late 1940s (following the formation of WHO) to roughly 1997/1998 (the beginnings of global public health emergency vigilance) as one of postcolonial outbreak communications. In the historian Sunil Amrith's words, WHO and other agencies in the UN system "were more consciously *inter-national* than the League of Nations, recognizing the primacy of the nation state as the appropriate agent for carrying out such policies [of disease control]" (Amrith 2006: 12).[3] Decolonization brought sovereignty to those formerly constituted as nonsovereign, but not equal sovereignty. During the 1950s and 1960s there was widespread discussion in the South about how to reform international law in order to remedy the wrongs of the colonial system and promote a new international order (Anghie 2007: 196–244).

Under the International Sanitary Regulations (International Sanitary Regulations [ISR] 1951) newly sovereign states in the Third World and former colonial powers were made equal under international health law. These Regulations were designed to prevent the international spread of infectious diseases under postcolonial conditions and were similar to previous international conventions in focusing on what were called "quarantinable" diseases. The quarantinable diseases in the ISR (1951) consisted of plague, cholera, yellow fever, smallpox, typhus, and relapsing fever. These diseases were made "notifiable" by national health administrations, which means that the country members of WHO were legally obligated to report all cases occurring in their territories (ISR 1951: Art. 3). Notifications (except for rodent plague) were to be followed by supplementary information about "the source and type of the disease, the number of cases and deaths, the conditions affecting the spread of the disease, and the prophylactic measures taken" (ISR 1951, Art. 4).

Each country member of WHO was legally obligated to report cases of quarantinable disease. Only sovereign states could legally report quarantinable diseases, and each sovereign state could only report those that occurred within its own territory. Whereas colonial administrations had distributed epidemiological information internationally through the Far Eastern Bureau, the ISR (1951) vested legal control of communicable disease information in the sovereign states that were WHO members. Notification under the ISR (1951) politically authorized WHO to have a knowledge of record; that is, WHO could notify its members or speak to the press about an outbreak/epidemic if and only if WHO had received an official report from the country member in question. Notification was thus a sovereign act, and we have chosen to refer to it sociologically as 'official,' in preference to the public health term 'formal,' in recognition of its political character as an act of state. We use the term 'unofficial,' in preference to 'informal,' to describe the many ways in which WHO knew and currently knows about outbreak and other public health events other than through official channels.

The ISR (1951) clearly articulated a legal standard for the timely official report of outbreak. Urgent communications were to be sent by telegram and nonurgent communications sent by airmail. Under conditions of quarantinable disease outbreak, health administrations were required to notify WHO "by telegram within twenty-four hours" (ISR 1951: Art. 3). The ISR

(1951) obligated WHO country members to send weekly reports by telegram that summarized the number of cases and deaths from a quarantinable disease close to a port or airport in their jurisdictions (ISR 1951: Art. 9). If no cases occurred in a given week, the national health administration was to send the report by airmail (ISR 1951: Art. 9). WHO was placed under a reciprocal obligation to communicate information promptly to its country members: "Communications of an urgent nature shall be sent by telegram or telephone" (ISR 1951: Art. 11). Under conditions of "exceptional emergency" involving a quarantinable disease, the telegrams and telephone calls of Member States and of WHO were to be given a priority that was "the highest available under international telecommunications agreements" (ISR 1951: Art. 12).

During the postcolonial period, WHO country members did not orient to the accelerated time demands that were later characteristic of global emergency vigilance. Although, as we will show in this and the following chapters, WHO officials were chronically impatient with the pace of epidemiological reporting under international health law during the postcolonial period, few country members of WHO were fundamentally discontented with the then-existing speed of epidemiological communications. One sees evidence of this patience in the country responses to two WHO surveys. The first survey occurred in 1946 and was ordered by the Interim Commission of WHO.[4] UN members were asked about the practical uses to which they put epidemiological intelligence and what they recommended for the future WHO epidemiological service. In the report of the 1946 survey, *An Enquiry into the Use Made by the Various Countries of the Epidemiological Intelligence Received from the WHO,*[5] 12 of 31 country member respondents replied there was a need for "speeding-up of transmission and dissemination of information";[6] that is, 19 of 31 respondents saw no need for increased speed. The second survey was an internal WHO evaluation done in 1971 of the Daily Epidemiological Radio Bulletin (DERB), which broadcasted urgent information about infectious disease outbreaks on a daily basis from WHO headquarters in Geneva between 1949 and 1972.[7] The 1971 survey of DERB's use (undertaken prior to its discontinuance and replacement by telex) established that few countries listened to it. Dr. Ian Carter, in a memorandum to Dr. E. Roelsgaard, Chief of Epidemiological Surveillance of Communicable Diseases, observed that "[t]heoretically the DERB may be of great value as a means of rapid transmission of communicable disease information but in practice at the present time it would appear to be monitored by the health administrators of only a few countries."[8] Carter then referred to the survey results showing that only 23 countries listened to the DERB, 14 of which were European. That the DERB had so few users was one of the reasons that justified WHO's move to telex.[9] Taken together the results of the 1946 and 1971 surveys indicate that only a minority of country members had an interest in speeding up the epidemiological communications they received from WHO.

Although postcolonial states asserted sovereign control over infectious disease information, the colonial legacy continued in public health as it did in politics, economics, and culture. The pattern of rupture and continuity in official epidemiological communications can be seen in DERB, which operated from Geneva (WHO 1958: 263, Map 2; see Fig. 3.1, p. 70). The DERB repeated the previous pattern of colonial communications in being organized primarily along a North-South axis, with a secondary pattern of lateral, East-West communications in Asia and the Western Pacific. Epidemiological communication was routed through the urban hubs of empire: Singapore, Alexandria (now Cairo), and Washington, DC, although Geneva displaced London, Paris, and Rome as the European metropole. Postcolonial surveillance occurred after imperial surveillance; it was continuous and discontinuous with the previous period.

Read in relation to international health law, only officially reported epidemiological knowledge appears present in the postcolonial period of international infectious disease control. However, WHO archival records show the importance of news reports for the work of WHO officials in communicable disease control throughout the second half of the 20th century. Registering the significance of news moves towards a more empirically sound understanding of the scale and form of its organizational presence in international disease surveillance.

During the postcolonial period official epidemiological communications existed in relation to a capacious other: unofficial knowledge, all those ways WHO knew about communicable disease outbreaks that were not authorized by the sovereign states in which the outbreak/epidemic was occurring or had occurred. News reports were a particularly significant form of unofficial outbreak information and were drawn upon as an unsystematic practical knowledge in the everyday work of public health authorities, functioning as a means to detect outbreak, often more quickly than through official channels. Unofficial knowledge, often sourced in newspaper reports, would precipitate official and nonofficial public health inquiries to confirm or disconfirm outbreak. In their work practices public health administrators attempted to coordinate and align official with unofficial knowledge. But when the country members of WHO delayed or refused to report outbreak, WHO personnel sometimes found themselves caught between sovereign states and the news media, excoriated by the press for incompetence. Under these conditions, when unofficial knowledge of outbreak met no official confirmation, the relation between official and unofficial knowledge became one of tension and conflict.

In the period from the 1950s to the mid-1990s, news was a source of unofficial practitioner knowledge of outbreak, one that was neither politically nor scientifically warranted. News was not recognized as a legitimate source for scientific epidemiology, which held itself to the normative standard of being sourced in clinical and laboratory diagnoses. Associated with 'rumor,' news became the antithesis of scientific surveillance. Yet

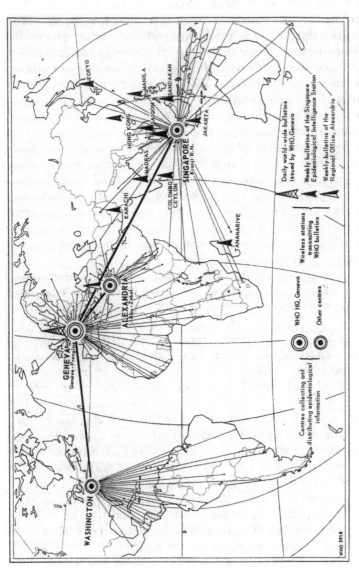

Figure 3.1   Network of epidemiological radio-telegraphic communications. Reprinted with permission of the World Health Organization.

Comment: The Daily Epidemiological Radio Bulletin (DERB) broadcasted urgent information about infectious disease outbreaks on a daily basis from WHO headquarters in Geneva between 1949 and 1972. The DERB network operated primarily on a North-South axis, thus repeating the prior spatial organization of colonial communications. A secondary pattern of lateral, East-West, communications was found in Asia and the Western Pacific.

Source: WHO 1958: 263, Map 2: Network of Epidemiological Radio-Telegraphic Communications. Reproduced with the permission of the World Health Organization.

news reports consistently informed public health action at WHO and the CDC during this period. Even during the high waters of case-based epidemiological surveillance at the CDC, news reports were part of surveillance efforts. Alexander Langmuir (1963: 188), who during the 1950s steered the development of epidemiological surveillance as a practice of collecting data on a population basis, recognized news as a component of the 1957 CDC influenza surveillance programme. After he noted that "[m]aintaining surveillance over a disease such as epidemic influenza involving up to tens of millions of cases on a national basis presented special statistical problems," Langmuir (1963: 188) stated that influenza surveillance included "more effective indexes" such as "simple narrative reports of epidemics and outbreaks" and "newspaper reports of the recognized prevalence of influenza in a city or a county as measured by closing of schools or increased absenteeism in industry."

Clippings from newspapers and references to news reports regularly appear in archived WHO administrative documents pertaining to communicable diseases. WHO used news as a source of information about outbreak and responded to the information in several ways. News reports alerted public health officials to underreporting of communicable disease cases and outbreaks. Formal and informal inquiries about outbreak were sometimes initiated by WHO personnel in response to news reports, and field investigations would on occasion be launched. WHO officials sometimes dealt with news reports of an outbreak by documenting their prior knowledge and actions to those in higher management positions in the organization. The most difficult situation for WHO with respect to news occurred when international press coverage alerted its country members to a likely outbreak but no official confirmation could be obtained.

Clippings of news reports about outbreaks and epidemics were forwarded to WHO headquarters in Geneva, often accompanying memoranda dealing with field investigations and aid during epidemics. The internal memoranda sometimes contained no reference to the clippings being forwarded with them, assuming that press coverage was of self-evident interest to those at WHO headquarters. One example of this textual practice can be seen in the appearance of a short article from *The Statesman*, "The Maldives' Ordeal by Cholera," amidst WHO correspondence related to the 1978 cholera epidemic in the Maldives.[10] At another point during this epidemic, a quite different use of news occurred when the International Monetary Fund, about to send a mission to the Maldives, requested clarifying information from WHO after reading an international news report from Reuters about cholera there: "imf, new york, informed me that imf mission is scheduled to arrive in Maldives next week. Report of cholera has been received thru reuters news agency. Imf would appreciate earliest information this epidemic."[11]

News reports of communicable disease outbreaks continually called WHO to account for its internal and external actions actions. Officials at

WHO headquarters in Geneva were sometimes forwarded news reports of an outbreak and reacted with internal memoranda that documented WHO health activities prior to and during the outbreak. The internal memoranda made visible to those higher up in the WHO bureaucracy work that had already occurred and that could be used, if necessary, to defend WHO's external actions. An instance of this scrupulous internal bureaucratic process can be seen in the memorandum of Dr. Paul Brès (Chief of Viral Diseases) to Dr. I.D. Ladnyi (Assistant Director-General) sent through Dr. A. Zahra (Director of the CDS, Division of Communicable Diseases), dated December 20, 1977, on the subject of "Rift Valley Fever Outbreak in Egypt."[12] The first sentence of this memorandum reads: "The attached information which was provided by Mr. Gino Levi, appeared in the Herald Tribune today."[13] Dr. Brès then remarked that his office had been aware of the outbreak as evidenced in his memoranda of November 7, 1977, and November 24, 1977, copies of which he attached. Further, Dr. Brès' office had both received and edited a report on the outbreak that had already been published in the *Weekly Epidemiological Record*. Finally, Dr. Brès concluded, a report by Dr. Robert Shope, Director of the WHO Collaborating Centre Arbovirus Reference and Research, had been commissioned. In forwarding the memorandum, Dr. A. Zahra, the Director of the CDS, added a short comment that the situation showed the need for country members, WHO Regional Offices, and staff to be more aware of and use the WHO's Aid in Epidemics programme. Thus an elaborate textual practice internal to WHO established that the organization had fulfilled its responsibilities and that it was indeed the responsibility of others to have requested aid. Three internal memoranda, one official publication, and one commissioned report defended WHO against one lone newspaper report of outbreak.

WHO officials sometimes followed the publication of news stories with various kinds of information gathering. Inquiries and field investigations were sometimes launched in response to press reports, as occurred during a 1987 outbreak of dengue fever in Jakarta. In March 1987, WHO headquarters in Geneva, the WHO Regional Office for South-East Asia, and the WHO Regional Office for the European and Mediterranean region requested information about an outbreak from the WHO office in Jakarta. The Jakarta office replied by a telegram that mentioned a field investigation that had followed a local news report: "The outbreak was reported in Jakarta press and was investigated stop there were seventyfour cases and nine deaths and outbreak is due to dengue haemorrhagic fever stop."[14] A press report provoked a field investigation in Italy after *Newsweek* magazine published an article about an outbreak of respiratory disease at a hospital in Naples during the period between 1978 and 1979. A field investigation of the outbreak[15] was instigated after members of the public who had read this news report asked the Italian government for clarification. WHO used news as a source of information about outbreak, but once the news of outbreak had spread in the local press, and particularly the international press, there existed time pressures on WHO to respond by demonstrating its control of the situation through the actions it had taken and/or displaying pertinent scientific information.

News articles could also be useful to WHO officials for identification of outbreaks that countries did not report. A 1977 letter from Ian Carter in Epidemiological Surveillance of Communicable Diseases, WHO headquarters, remarked that "[t]he newspaper reports related to the number of cases in Indonesia has not been reflected in the official notifications from the national health administration."[16] Country members' underreporting of notifiable communicable diseases was a common problem for WHO public health officials, but when news reports called attention to an outbreak that had not been confirmed by a country member, WHO was placed in the potentially difficult situation of seeming to know less about public health than the press did, and being unable to confirm or disconfirm an outbreak both to the media and to its own country members. A 1987 communication from the WHO Regional Office for Africa to the WHO country office in Algeria contains a clipping with the title "Algerian Silence about Cholera Outbreak" from *World Water*, together with a French translation of that article, and a covering memorandum pointedly requesting that the country office call the attention of the relevant Algerian parties to the article and remind them of WHO's role should a problem arise.[17] Another case of the press outpacing WHO occurred in 1985 when WHO Director-General Hans Mahler made an official diplomatic request for confirmation of a cholera outbreak to the Minister of Health, Addis Ababa, Ethiopia: "[d]istressed by repeated newspaper reports describing outbreaks of alleged cholera in Ethiopia primarily in refugee camps. Whether or not such reports are true, they are confusing and lead to misunderstanding."[18] In this passage, WHO is situated as a reader of "repeated" news reports that undermined the alignment between WHO and its country member, Ethiopia. The WHO Director-General's appeal to the Minister of Health of Ethiopia for an official country communication was intended to restore the relation between WHO and its country member, a relation that was being undermined by press reports. Information about outbreak in this case was controlled neither by WHO nor by the government of Ethiopia.

News had the capacity to circulate information about communicable disease outbreaks that was critical of WHO and its country members, making each seem to be either secretive or ignorant. One might call this a news strategy of shame, which is present under conditions where rival social actors compete for symbolic recognition in terms of a particular expertise. The practice of shaming involves a social actor's upstaging another actor's authorized expertise. Shame is a strategy of the public sphere for undermining those in power who are presented as incompetent. Operating through oral and written speech, shame potentially damages the social recognition given expertise unless those being discredited can respond by finding some means to reaffirm their symbolic worth. Shame does damage to what Bourdieu (1984: 291) calls the symbolic capital of professionals: "a reputation for competence and an image of respectability and honourability."

The strategy of shame was used by the press against WHO during the major outbreak of cholera in Guinea that occurred during 1970, where, for the only time in the history of the International Health Regulations (1969), WHO reported an outbreak to its members and the international press without prior country confirmation (Fidler 2004b: 64–65). The history of this outbreak is well known (Fidler 2004b: 64–65; Leive 1976: 82–85), but the significance of the press in establishing the crisis conditions for the WHO Director-General to act in violation of the International Health Regulations has not been investigated or conceptualized. Despite repeated requests from the WHO Director-General, who had received reliable information from nongovernmental sources, the government of Guinea did not confirm that a cholera epidemic was occurring within its borders, although under the IHR (1969) all WHO country members had a duty to notify WHO of cholera within 24 hours of a case report. As cholera spread in Africa and the Middle East, countries were subjected to precautionary measures in excess of those mandated by the IHR.[19]

In a telex of August 28, 1970 to WHO Director-General Maurice Candau, Deputy Director-General Pierre Dorolle emphasized that the press was presenting an image of WHO as having done little about the epidemic in Guinea: "[u]nder increasing pressure from various sources governmental and others for information on real cholera situation and in view of the critical comments from world press on alleged inertia."[20] On that same day Dr. Dorolle sent a second telex to Dr. Candau suggesting that WHO consider broadcasting news of the outbreak in contravention of the IHR (1969): "[s]imilar cable would be dispatched Guinea if no reply within 48 hours to my first cable urging declare their cases stop segundo studying with all concerned including legal possibility broadcast information outside international regulations on basis information obtained from reliable sources stop shall consult before acting."[21] WHO had been placed in a position of knowing a great deal about the epidemic in Guinea but was unable to broadcast its activities to the press or confirm the outbreak with its country members.

WHO received official communications from its country members requesting clarification of the cholera epidemic in Guinea, with the French and U.S. letters noting the gap between newspaper reports and the information they were receiving from WHO:

> Le Gouvernement français fait part à l'Organisation mondiale de la Santé de sa préoccupation en ce qui concerne les divergences existant entre les informations sanitaires diffusées actuellement par les journaux et les renseignements donnés par l'Organisation mondiale de la Santé.[22] [The French government shares its concern with the World

Health Organization about discrepancies between the health information currently being provided by newspapers and the information distributed by the World Health Organization.]

I am greatly concerned with fact WHO not disclosing information on occurrence of Cholera in different countries, even with public press reporting in detail. I urge you to report to member governments all information on occurrence of Cholera reaching you from reliable sources.[23]

Not only was WHO shamed by the world press, but its country members were as well. Internal pressure from its country members then led WHO to violate the International Health Regulations. Replying to the letter from the U.S. Surgeon General (quoted in the second citation in preceding text), the WHO Director-General responded that he "shares the concern of Surgeon General and has come to conclusion that in absence of official notification from governments there is now no alternative but to disclose reliable information after final appeal to countries concerned. This is being done and the daily epidemiological broadcast of 1 September will contain relevant information."[24] In the aftermath of WHO's broadcast of information about the cholera epidemic in Guinea without official country confirmation, several Member States threatened to resign from WHO, with the result that WHO never again broadcasted a report of outbreak on the basis of unofficial information during the period in which the IHR (1969) was in effect. One isolated and poignant news clipping has been inserted without comment in the WHO archival record about the 1970 cholera epidemic in Guinea, an editorial from the *New York Times*, "Cholera and Politics," that defended WHO for having released information about the epidemic in Guinea and chid Guinean officials for their furious reaction.[25]

This account of the 1970 cholera epidemic in Guinea has emphasized that conflict over the control of report was not simply a dyadic one between WHO and its sovereign country members. Rather, the 1970 conflict was triangular and consisted of WHO, sovereign states, and the press. The resolution of the conflict should not be understood solely as the triumph of state sovereignty over international public health, but also as a demonstration of the effects of the press on international public health, where the press operated as a social actor capable of disseminating news of outbreak independently of WHO and its country members. The press was strategically capable of shaming both WHO and its country members under the legal conditions that obtained under the IHR (1969).

WHO not only responded to news of outbreak, but was also itself a source of news for the world press. By the early 1980s WHO was explicitly formulating a press policy for its work with the media under conditions of epidemic. A WHO report from an informal consultation in 1981 noted the difficulties that the WHO "unit of Information" experienced with unconfirmed reports of epidemic, which sometimes left WHO caught in "a time-lag between first press reports and confirmation or denial from official sources."[26] In this report, WHO perceived itself as caught in the middle, dealing with "a delay on the one hand of response from authorities, and impatience on the other on the part of the media."[27] Situations such as the one that had obtained with the Guinean government in 1970 bore special mention in the consultation report: "[m]ost trying of all are situations in which epidemics are known to be in progress, despite official denials formally transmitted to the WHO."[28] The 1981 consultation acknowledged that the media had easy access to news of outbreak, communicating it worldwide.[29] The position of WHO, it was argued, should be to improve press accuracy and reliability, to enlist the media in health promotion, and during epidemics to transmit public health recommendations, many of which had significance for economic stabilization in business, trade, and tourism.[30]

From this descriptive account of the relation between news and WHO in the postcolonial period of epidemiological communications, one can see that WHO entered into differing social relations with news. To WHO, news was in part a source of information about outbreak that often occurred prior to official confirmation. WHO responded to the disjunction between unofficial, news-based knowledge of outbreak and official knowledge of outbreak through a series of practices: launching unofficial and official inquiries, facilitating other organizations or itself to undertake field investigations, and in one disastrous case never repeated, announcing outbreak without country confirmation. WHO thus had a deeply ambivalent relation to news as, on the one hand, news reports were a valuable source of information about outbreak, while on the other hand, they entered into competition with the expertise of WHO, threatening it with symbolic damage. News formed a powerful rival on which international health authorities were dependent for knowledge of outbreak.

One can make a number of initial observations from this evidence. First, WHO nonofficial knowledge of outbreak/epidemic did exist in the period prior to the invention of early warning outbreak detection. Nonofficial knowledge was an unsystematic practical knowledge learned on the job in public health rather than a formal part of public health training. We have shown that international public health officials at WHO did not solely depend on official notifications by its country members for knowledge of outbreak. Their knowledge took two forms, official and unofficial. Only official report of outbreak became a knowledge of record; that is, information gathered by WHO in accordance with procedures specified under international health law could be publicly communicated. Second, the sources of unofficial knowledge, such as news reports, circulated transnationally outside sovereign control. Whereas official knowledge had a single source—the sovereign states that were the country members of the WHO—unofficial knowledge of outbreak had multiple sources. News of outbreak routed around national control to

connect international public health officials with local knowledge of outbreak. Official knowledge of outbreak was characterized by national control, linking local outbreak with international knowledge through a path
mandated in international public health law. The spatial organization of
news as an unofficial knowledge crossed the politico-spatial boundaries of
official knowledge. Third, unofficial knowledge frequently circulated faster
than official knowledge. Fourth, the relations between the two knowledge
forms, official and unofficial, were interactive and in competition. Because
international public health authorities at WHO were required to advise
country members about international outbreaks and epidemics, a field of
tensions existed between official and unofficial knowledge of outbreak.

Online Early Warning Outbreak Detection and Alert

By the mid-1990s WHO's system for knowing about and responding to
infectious disease outbreaks was decisively problematized by the global
North's demands for protection against EID. The detection and containment
of EID challenged the knowledge relations of postcolonial communicable
disease control, a challenge linked to demands for a form of international
epidemiological surveillance that would give WHO knowledge of domestic
infectious disease outbreaks while they were occurring. Over the course of
the 10-year revision process of the IHR (1969) between 1995 and 2005,
the objectives of public health surveillance at WHO were extended beyond
infectious disease control to include all international emergencies with a
public health component. The new form of surveillance that was expected
to detect so much and so quickly was termed 'online early warning outbreak detection.' The relations and tensions that characterized official and
unofficial international public health knowledge of outbreak in the period
from the 1950s to the late 1990s were redrawn under the impact of early
warning outbreak detection.

Early warning outbreak detection is a novel concept used in public
health to refer to recent innovations in the processes used to identify disease outbreaks and other events that are of international public health concern. These developments were propelled by a shift in understanding of the
microbial world as one subject to ongoing transformation, most dramatically manifested by the emergence of previously unknown infectious diseases. These developments were also driven by a growing recognition that
significant changes in conditions of global communication, particularly the
rise of electronic media, had not been sufficiently incorporated into established methods of international infectious disease detection and response
(Heymann et al. 2001).

Public health officials at WHO began writing about early warning outbreak detection in the late 1990s. They produced a series of articles that
positioned WHO as an innovator in the field, describing WHO's efforts to

revitalize international mechanisms for detecting and responding to outbreak through, for example, the invention of new forms of outbreak verification and the establishment of the Global Outbreak Alert and Response Network (Heymann & Rodier 1998; Grein et al. 2000: Heymann et al.; Rodier 2001). More recently, attention has been turned to a wide range of initiatives in early warning outbreak detection that operate within as well as beyond the formal orbit of the WHO system. Characteristic among these initiatives is an emphasis on the need to respond to a changed context of global public health risk by linking Web-based electronic information with established epidemiological sources of outbreak information (Paquet, Coulombier, Kaiser, & Ciotti 2006; Brownstein, Freifeld, Reis, & Mandl 2008; Hitchcock, Chamberlain, Van Wagoner, Inglesby, & O'Toole 2007; M'ikanatha, Lynfield, Van Beneden, & de Valk 2007).

The many initiatives that currently exist for early warning outbreak detection are carried forward through a set of relations linking microbial phenomena, human actors, organizations, information sources, computer technologies, and various forms of expertise in multiple ways. The organizational complex of these initiatives takes the form of networks that span hospital personnel and other health workers, epidemiologists and public health officials, national health departments, research institutes, public health and other Websites, news media, news aggregators, international health organizations, the CDC, and WHO, amongst others. The formation of this governance apparatus network required a revision of international health law and, as we will show in Chapter 5, the constitution of a suprasovereign political level in international health.

Early warning outbreak detection is in part a proxy method used to identify outbreaks under conditions wherein some national surveillance and response systems are regarded as weak—a weakness that may indicate other health system priorities such as directing funding to primary health care, which is the case, by way of example, in Cuba and Kerala. The present time is characterized by what is sometimes called a 'surveillance gap' between North and South. Support for the development of surveillance and response capacity in the South is a key political question that has arisen since the passage of the IHR (2005; *PLoS Medicine* Editors 2007; see also Chapter 4 for further discussion).

In this chapter we focus on the institutional architecture of early warning outbreak detection and alert that has been consolidated as part of the vigilance apparatus centered on the global public health security work of WHO. That architecture involves a sequence of activities that orients to containment of outbreaks and other emergencies by identifying and intervening in them as quickly as possible. The sequence begins with outbreak detection through which information about potential emergencies is communicated to WHO on the basis of official information but also, increasingly, via news and other types of unofficial information such as reports from nongovernmental organizations (Heymann et al. 2001). The sequence

proceeds to outbreak verification, a process coordinated by WHO to confirm outbreaks and substantiate that reported events are genuine international public health concerns (Grein et al. 2000). It ends with outbreak
alert and response, which involves the deployment of rapid response teams
to local sites of outbreak/emergency in order to contain these and prevent their spread. Our discussion here focuses on the first two parts of the
sequence: outbreak detection and verification.

A) Outbreak Detection

WHO currently receives unofficial information about infectious disease
outbreaks and related public health events from a number of sources:
nongovernmental organizations such as Médecins sans Frontières and
the Red Cross, Christian relief organizations, and various regional electronic mail-based discussion groups (Grein et al. 2000). The two most
important sources of informal, unofficial reports to WHO are GPHIN
and ProMED-mail, each of which are early warning outbreak detection
systems based on unofficial information. WHO data for 2001 to 2005
indicate that over 60% of reports of unverified outbreaks reported to the
WHO originated in unofficial sources of information, the majority from
GPHIN (Heymann 2006; Mawudeku, Lemay, Werker, Andraghetti, & St.
John 2007). Between 2001 and 2008 GPHIN supplied WHO with 2,415
alerts that were subsequently verified (Institute of Medicine and National
Research Council 2008: 55, Table 4–1). For the period January 1, 1998,
to December 31, 2005 (excluding data related to SARS and incomplete
information), WHO figures indicate that of 1,697 unverified events identified to be of potential international public health significance, 1,256 were
verified. Of these 1,256 verified events, 518 (41%) were from news sources,
and of these, GPHIN had major responsibility for 81% (422 of 518 verified
events) (Mawudeku et al. 2007: 310–311).

GPHIN is WHO's primary source of unofficial outbreak information.
It is best thought of as a secure, Internet-based global monitoring system for early detection of infectious disease outbreaks and related public
health events. The initiative was formally launched by Health Canada in
1998 and was developed in close collaboration with WHO. GPHIN is currently housed in the Centre for Emergency Preparedness and Response of
the Public Health Agency of Canada. The annual operating, upgrade, and
development costs of GPHIN are approximately CDN$3.5 million per year
(Mawudeku et al. 2007) and the activities of its 14 staff members are over-
seen by a manager.

The significance of online health news, both as a potential resource for
international infectious disease control and as a threat to the credibility of
WHO's international system of outbreak notification that historically relied
on official country reporting of infectious disease outbreaks, features promi-
nently in accounts of the development of GPHIN. The public health officials

responsible for creating GPHIN began imagining its form and potential in the early 1990s at a time that roughly coincided with the publication of the early reports on EID described in the previous chapter and the calls those reports generated for enhanced global health surveillance. The originators of GPHIN concluded early on that improvements in the speed and breadth of international infectious disease surveillance would require moving beyond epidemiological case reports and official country notification.

The timeliness of notification under the existent arrangements was a central concern for GPHIN's founders. One GPHIN interview participant noted that the volume and increased speed of international air travel posed significant challenges to traditional methods of epidemiological surveillance. International travel by airplane meant that passengers crossed national borders well within incubation periods and before the appearance of clinical symptoms. The compression of travel time associated with the shift of international travel from ships to airplanes required approaches to the detection of infectious diseases that were faster than those relying on epidemiological confirmation of clinical cases.

The delays associated with the formal system of international infectious disease control established and coordinated by WHO was also a concern. As mentioned before and discussed in greater detail in Chapter 4, at the time of our GPHIN interviews, that system was coordinated by the IHR (1969), which legally authorized sovereign control over the report of outbreaks occurring within national territories. Under the terms of the IHR (1969), WHO could only take public action in response to infectious disease outbreaks on the basis of official country reports, and country members were only required to report outbreaks of plague, yellow fever, cholera and, before its eradication, small pox. In speaking about this system, one GPHIN interview participant used the common epidemiological term 'passive surveillance' to refer to its inherent communication limitations:

> I should back up and say that the system that was in place for years and decades is a kind of passive surveillance system. The local area in a country is expected to report to some kind of regional area health district, and they're supposed to report up to the national government; and then the national government, if they so elect, will contact WHO ... The WHO had to be very passive about that for political reasons. Although offline there would be insistence that the country please report, so that WHO could say something about it, that could be on relatively frequent occasions ignored by the countries. (GPHIN Interview)

The research participant calls the official system of notification that existed at WHO a "kind of passive surveillance system" that was accompanied by "offline" inquiries.[31] In passive surveillance systems, public health authorities wait for case reports to be communicated to them; the reports are for diseases and conditions mandated by law and in public health regulations.

The many critiques of WHO's system of international infectious disease control were well known to the originators of GPHIN. As previously noted, countries were routinely noncompliant with the notification terms of the IHR (1969). The economic repercussions of reporting, particularly the prospect of dramatic losses in travel and trade, often meant that countries delayed reporting or chose not to report at all (Cash & Narasimhan 2000). The system also contained no provisions for reporting EID, the popularization of which had been behind the call to revise the existent system of international infectious disease surveillance. While calling the pre-1998 WHO system of communicable disease identification passive surveillance underestimates its active elements, "passive surveillance" nevertheless captured for our GPHIN research participants the central, immediate problem of international infectious disease reporting: incomplete and delayed notification. Reflecting on reports that were often months (if not years) overdue, one GPHIN official noted that while they might prove useful for future prevention work, they were of no value for responding to reported outbreaks.

For the originators of GPHIN, a newfound awareness of the role played by news in the public circulation of unofficial knowledge about infectious diseases outbreaks was decisive for moving from a critique of the existent system of international infectious disease surveillance to imagining an alternative that responded to its central weaknesses. The pivotal moment was the outbreak of pneumonic plague in Surat, India, in 1994.

The Surat outbreak was among the first infectious disease outbreaks to obtain widespread, near real-time global news coverage. The Surat epidemic received international publicity through established international newswire services such as Reuters, through radio channels such as the BBC, and through the newer form of global portable satellite television such as CNN International, which had been established in 1985 to cover global news on a 24-hour, 7 days a week basis (Medina 2003: 85). CNN International's coverage included footage of people fleeing the city. Newspapers in major urban centers across the world, including the global North, ran stories about the outbreak under such headlines as the following: "Indians Panic Over Plague—200,000 Flee City Where Disease Has Killed at Least 24,"[32] "Medical Experts Fear Refugees May Spread India Plague" (Burns 1994), and "Red Alert in Bombay and New Delhi as Plague Fear Shifts to More Indian Cities" (Rettie 1994). Media coverage of the Surat outbreak is widely recognized to have generated unprecedented global panic about an epidemic. One of our interview participants described its manifestation in the Canadian context:

And there were pictures of people fleeing the city on CNN. And we were watching that and of course that immediately gave rise to some anxiety in Canada because we have such a large Indian community and we have so much travel between the two countries. Even to the point where . . . we recognized that there was already a flight en route to

Toronto by Air India, and it threatened work stoppage at the Pearson
Airport because this plane might be hauling plague . . . So we tried to
monitor this thing. (GPHIN Interview)

Subsequent commentary has criticized the role of the global media in fanning
public anxieties about an outbreak that lasted only 2 weeks and in which fewer
than 1,200 individuals were diagnosed (Dutt, Akhtar, & McVeigh 2006).
From the perspective of the founders of GPHIN, however, what was particularly striking at the time was how their own monitoring efforts were being
triggered not by official notifications received through WHO channels but
through public news reports of the outbreak. The Indian government initially
refused to acknowledge the outbreak and delayed notifying WHO; the earliest
reports that an outbreak had occurred originated in global health news.

Critical accounts of media-generated panic point to important ways in
which news shapes responses to infectious disease outbreak, often with
devastating economic consequences for host countries. But they leave aside
the less dramatic ways that news coverage has been consequential for international public health detection of and response to infectious disease. The
outbreak in Surat was an important example of how the pace of unofficial
news coverage eclipsed the cumbersome routes of official WHO outbreak
notification. News was more important for early public health monitoring
and response to the outbreak in Surat than WHO official reports, if only
because WHO handled its news coverage from Geneva rather than the government of India. WHO announced the formation of an international field
team on Oct. 7, 1994, reporting on Dec. 9, 1994 (WHO 1994: 277). As the
highest mortality occurred between September 20 and September 24 (Shah
1997: 220), WHO arrived very much after the fact. Satellite TV had created
information about the outbreak faster and had generated responses well
before epidemiological communications had been officially communicated
by India. News challenged WHO's claims to know about local outbreaks
and displaced formal notifications as the primary mode of communication
and basis of global public health response to the outbreak:

> Countries started to do some strange things, like ban their ships going
> to India. The towns put doctors on their airplanes to monitor whether
> or not there was any coughing on board the plane, I mean there were
> some really strange things that happened. And we were trying to moni-
> tor all this. We were trying to get information from WHO. At that time
> WHO basically went home on the weekends . . . What was actually
> happening was that the media was so far ahead of the health sector in
> monitoring and reporting . . . that the media was driving the reaction,
> not the World Health Organization. (GPHIN Interview)

This interview participant presents an institutional disjuncture between
monitoring and reporting by WHO and the news media. The result was

a public relations disaster for WHO at a point when it was being openly questioned as inefficient and inept (Kickbusch 2000: 983).

With respect to WHO, the Surat outbreak of 1994 was a specific kind of disaster—a temporal one. News problematized the temporal relations of how infectious disease outbreaks came into knowledge in public health. Global satellite television constituted the 1994 plague in Surat as what Virilio has called a "global accident"/global media event constituted by live coverage watched on every continent. The international news media inserted Surat into a synchronized global time, whereas outbreaks previously had been inscribed in local and/or national time. Virilio's words give historical insight into the formation of a global time as distinct from national and local time: "All of history was inscribed in local time, in local space and time. Time in China is not the same as time in Europe, just as time in Paris is not time in Aix-en-Provence, and so on. Now the history that is beginning is synchronized to world time, in other words, it's happening 'live'" (Virilio 1997: 185). WHO's actions in 1994 assumed the outbreak in Surat had the same temporal organization that had characterized outbreaks since the beginning of WHO's international communicable disease under the ISR (1951); the time of outbreak had generally been local with weak links to national and international temporal orders. But satellite news had changed the temporal organization of outbreak unbeknownst to national and international public health. The remedy required a technique that would accelerate public health knowledge, one that would bring public health knowledge of outbreak into synchronized world time. One might say that such a technique would bring public health up to speed, but the question is precisely which speed and whose time.

During the Surat outbreak the founders of GPHIN established e-mail contact with a physician based in Surat and began an e-mail correspondence with him about the numbers of new patients being admitted to the hospital at which he worked. The string of communications they produced—a series of e-mail posts based on firsthand reports—was very much in keeping with the model of outbreak detection subsequently developed by the Listserv ProMED-mail, which we discuss later in this chapter. The use of news coverage and e-mail by GPHIN's founders to monitor the Surat plague pointed to new possibilities for the types of knowledge that might be legitimately drawn upon in early detection of disease outbreaks:

> All of a sudden it dawned on myself and another gentleman here that we had information the government and media didn't have, and it was all sort of informal. And it occurred to us that maybe the world was changing and that maybe there were other ways to get information besides waiting for the government. (GPHIN Interview)

There followed a period of considering various alternatives that might instrumentalize the possible uses of official knowledge in a novel system of outbreak detection, including an assessment of the approach being developed by ProMED-mail. In the end, the originators of GPHIN chose to pursue a system based on monitoring electronic news sources rather than one designed around an e-mail Listserv, like ProMED-mail. The latter was considered too reactive in that its design meant "waiting for people to go out and post things" and too slow, given that reports could not be released until after they had gone through an internal review process. After initial thoughts to develop a search engine that would crawl the World Wide Web proved unfeasible due technological limitations and the ever-growing size of the Web, the creators of GPHIN set their sights on harnessing electronic text-mining strategies that, as one research participant put it, "could handle text as though it were data." Such strategies would be applied to information procured from electronic news aggregators. What resulted was a remarkable moment of innovation in global public health in which complex, automated strategies for searching electronic words and relationships among them were used to identify potentially relevant news information and enter it into new uses within an emerging system of global public health vigilance.

The development of GPHIN occurred in the Canadian context. Leading research on automatic translation has been done in Canada, which is an officially bilingual country. In particular, research done in Quebec at the Université de Montréal, Département de linguistique et de traduction, was part of an international effort that began in the late 1980s to automatically detect terms found in computerized texts (Castellvi, Bagot, & Palatresi 2001: 53). New technologies for information and communication such as the Internet created an increased volume of texts that were identified as needing review for many differing organizational purposes (Rousseau & Depecker 1999: 2); these purposes included those of computer engineers, translators, linguists, science journalists, and departments of state. Software was invented to extract terminology from computerized texts, particularly through the development of taxonomies such as "building glossaries, vocabularies, and terminological dictionaries; text indexing; automatic translation; building of knowledge databases; construction of hypertext systems; construction of expert systems and corpus analysis" (Castellvi, Bagot, & Palatresi 2001: 53). GPHIN drew on this automatic term detection and translation capacity, adapting it for public health purposes.

The work of developing GPHIN began in earnest after funding was secured from a 1996 Canadian Federal Treasury Board competition for new initiatives using the Internet. The first version of GPHIN—the GPHIN prototype system—became operational in 1998 as part of a series of pilot projects created under Canada's National Health Surveillance Infostructure (Mawudeku et al. 2007). The pilot projects were intended to "demonstrate the use of the Internet for accessing and exchanging health surveillance information" (Health Surveillance Working Group 2003, cited in Mawudeku et al. 2007: 304). The purpose of the GPHIN prototype system was to explore the feasibility of using electronic news media reports for early warning outbreak detection and, if the same was found to be feasible, to establish a technology and infrastructure for developing an early warning system based on global news media (Mawudeku et al. 2007). A second version of GPHIN was formally launched in November 2004. Whereas the GPHIN prototype searched online news articles in French and English, the second version was multilingual and required search and automated translation modifications to handle a larger volume of news reports. The GPHIN multilingual system operates in English, French, Spanish, Portuguese, Russian, Arabic, Chinese (simplified and traditional), and Farsi and was developed through a research collaboration agreement with Nstein Technologies, a Montreal-based firm that markets multilingual online content management and text-mining solutions.

The majority of raw information that the GPHIN system scans takes the form of online news reports supplied by two news aggregators: Factiva and Al Bawaba. The GPHIN platform automatically scans these sources every 15 minutes across a number of topic areas: animal diseases, human diseases, plant diseases, biologics, natural disasters, chemical incidents, radioactive incidents, and unsafe products (Mawudeku & Blench 2006). In order to focus the scanning process on reports of greatest potential relevance, GPHIN uses an automated scanning system that is built around a custom-made taxonomy and search syntax. The taxonomy and search syntax are key forms of intellectual property closely guarded by GPHIN. They consist of a host of keywords and associated search syntaxes (word combinations and spacings between words) that are all modified for the different languages in which GPHIN searches and that are all subject to continual modification.

The GPHIN system scans roughly 20,000 sources of information in the languages in which it operates. On any given day, roughly 2,000 news items are processed; when the media covers a public health event that has captured global attention, that number easily doubles (GPHIN Interview). The scanning system filters out duplicates and gives relevancy scores to news items on the basis of values assigned to keywords and terms that appear in the news report and in GPHIN's taxonomy (Mawudeku et al. 2007). The system treats as irrelevant news items that have a relevancy score of 30 or less. These items are not available for viewing on the system by users but are kept in the GPHIN database. Items with a relevancy score between 30 and 85 are reviewed by GPHIN analysts before being posted to the GPHIN database for users to view. Reports with a score higher than 85 are immediately posted for GPHIN users to view (Mawudeku et al. 2007).

GPHIN's automated scanning, filtering, and categorizing processes are supplemented by the work of a team of multilingual human analysts with knowledge of current international infectious disease trends and the broader political and economic context of regions from which reports of potential outbreaks have occurred. GPHIN analysts also have expertise in a variety of disciplines including public health, medicine, biology, chemistry, environmental science, and journalism (Mawudeku et al. 2007). GPHIN's automated translation capacities provide 'gisted' translations of English articles into the system's other eight languages as well as gisted translations of non-English articles into English. Gisted translations are intended to summarize a news report and are generated by automated software. An algorithm assigns a comprehensibility score to gisted translations; those below a certain threshold are reviewed and enhanced by GPHIN analysts (Mawudeku & Blench 2006; Mawudeku et al. 2007: 306). GPHIN analysts flag roughly one to two news items per day as alerts. News items are categorized as alerts on the basis of the criteria set out by the IHR (2005) for determining if an event may constitute a public health emergency of international concern. Copies of the reports flagged as alerts are electronically sent to WHO and all other GPHIN users, which currently number approximately 150 (as of February 2009). All other news items with the required relevancy score are viewable by GPHIN users "through a password-protected interface anywhere there is Internet access" (Mawudeku 2007: 308). Users are able to view processed news reports in any of the languages in which GPHIN operates and can also prioritize the information they view by establishing a system of folders, each of which corresponds to a particular topic or region of interest (GPHIN Interview). GPHIN analysts are electronically available to users to address questions related to specific reports. GPHIN analysts also post special reports that add additional levels of analysis to individual news items. Special reports may offer summaries or updates on a specific issue of current global public health interest, including information on the scope and geographical distribution of the event or the public health measures being taken in response to it (GPHIN Interview).

The majority of GPHIN's users are public health organizations concerned with infectious disease outbreaks. These include disease control centers, public health departments, and ministries of health. Like ProMED-mail, however, GPHIN has a complex relationship to the deliberate spread of pathogens. The multiple functionality of GPHIN, its capacity to identify potential deliberately caused outbreaks, and the flexibility of its search strategy to meet the needs of multiple users have created interest in GPHIN amongst national defense departments. Faced with chronic underfunding for the ongoing enhancement and development of the GPHIN system, GPHIN moved to a cost-recovery model in September 2004 through which users are charged subscription fees and services are tailored to meet individual client needs.[33] Among the specialized services GPHIN offers is the early detection of bioterrorist events of interest to military intelligence. GPHIN's potential use by military clients and its need to secure additional revenues through subscription fees posed problems for WHO's diplomatic neutrality and were among the factors that transformed a formal collaboration with WHO into a client relationship.

The entry into force of the IHR (2005) in June 2007 has introduced important changes to the scope of GPHIN's operations. At a national level, Canada's efforts to fulfill new core capacities in domestic surveillance and response required by the IHR (2005) have expedited a reassessment of the utility of GPHIN and secured for it a new organizational role and stability within the Public Health Agency of Canada (PHAC).[34] In response to the IHR (2005), PHAC has created new program areas with responsibilities for intelligence gathering, risk assessment, and response capacity. GPHIN is now located within PHAC's Health Portfolio Operations Centre and has strengthened its surveillance capacities in order to conduct expanded detection and assessment of public health risks of concern to Canada. As part of its new service role within PHAC, in addition to its regular search functions, GPHIN now routinely monitors information from other sources such as Ministry of Health Web sites, regulatory institutions, and the IHR Web site, and reports information on events of concern to Canada in daily meetings with PHAC officials. Recognizing the strategic value of GPHIN for meeting IHR (2005) requirements, PHAC management has committed CDN$1.5 million per year to the GPHIN budget and is continuing to determine the most appropriate financial strategy to secure long-term and adequate funding for the GPHIN program. The financial insecurity that was part of GPHIN's past has been replaced by a renewed commitment to GPHIN by the Canadian government. Most recently, for example, PHAC has doubled the number of GPHIN analysts to 14.

At an international level, GPHIN has begun to play a stronger role in efforts to facilitate communication across different early warning outbreak systems. The vision of a 'world on alert' that grounds the IHR (2005) requires that outbreak information be rapidly and easily shared across the globe. However, a common platform enabling interaction across early warning systems does not yet exist. GPHIN is participating in a pilot project to create such a platform under the leadership of the Global Health Security Initiative, an informal partnership linking health ministries from the G8 countries, Mexico, and the European Union.

GPHIN is an important site of innovation in global public health practice. It has developed methods of outbreak detection that respond to the monitoring demands of global public health vigilance and EID. GPHIN has created the conditions that make possible the systematic treatment of news as an information base for detecting disease outbreaks and related public health events internationally. GPHIN's use of online sources and its application of electronic text-mining strategies, automated translation, and human expertise have the effect of rerouting health news into new institutional uses. GPHIN has created a set of techniques through which health news that is initially produced for public consumption, information, and entertainment is identified, modified, and inserted into the institutional relevancies of global public health, where it helps coordinate new relations of outbreak detection and alert.

The speed with which GPHIN accomplishes this is unprecedented. The SARS outbreak is an often-noted example of the quickness of the GPHIN system's detection capabilities. While ProMED-mail claims to have *publicly* distributed the first report of the SARS outbreak, GPHIN officials are quick to note that the first report of SARS was issued by GPHIN on November 27, 2002 (Mawudeku & Blench 2006). The report, in Chinese with a heading translated into English, did not mention SARS (a term that had not yet been invented at that point) but described unusual increases in emergency room visits in Guangdong, China. A subsequent report in English issued on January 21, 2003 once again did not mention an outbreak but described unusual increases in antiviral drug sales by a pharmaceutical company based in Guangdong. GPHIN's first report was issued roughly 3 months prior to the formal announcement of the SARS outbreak by WHO. GPHIN's outbreak reporting on SARS is widely recognized to have played a key role in WHO's efforts to secure verification of the outbreak from China (Heymann 2006).

The second official information source included in our discussion, ProMED-mail, was launched in 1994 as the communication system of the Program for Monitoring Emerging Diseases (ProMED). ProMED was founded in 1993 at a conference cosponsored by the Federation of American Scientists[35] and WHO that was attended by "60 prominent health experts from all parts of the world" to promote the "establishment of a global Program to Monitor Emerging Diseases" (Morse, Rosenberg, & Woodall 1996: 136, 135). ProMED sought to establish a demonstration project consisting of a network of institutions based primarily in developing countries that would be linked one with another and with local and regional organizations to monitor a "limited number of defined syndromes" (Morse et al. 1996: 135). While the full institutional network envisaged by ProMED never became fully operational, ProMED-mail, the planned electronic communication system for the network, did.

ProMED-mail was initiated at a second ProMED conference held in 1994. At that time some 40 conference participants joined an e-mail list for the purpose of maintaining contact with one another and sharing information on outbreak. The list was named ProMED-mail. ProMED-mail was the first ever global Internet network established for the purpose of exchanging unofficial information on infectious disease outbreaks. The originators of ProMED-mail responded to the demand for faster information on infectious disease outbreaks by harnessing the near real-time communication properties of the Internet, particularly e-mail. The vision was to use the low-cost, publicly available technology of e-mail to link individuals globally, to do so independently of government and other formal organizational channels, and to quickly exchange information on local outbreaks (Madoff & Woodall 2005). From the outset, ProMED-mail has focused on threats to human health posed by emerging infectious diseases amongst humans, animals, and plants, including threats related to their potential use for bioterrorism. ProMED-mail currently operates in English, Spanish, Portuguese, and French. The initiative is structured around a publicly accessible Web site (www.promedmail.com) where reports of outbreaks are posted and a variety of moderated e-mail Listservs with a combined membership of over 40,000 subscribers in approximately 165 countries.[36] ProMED-mail offers access to its Website and Listservs at no cost to users (Woodall 1997).

ProMED-mail issues approximately seven reports daily, 365 days per year. These reports are generated from two major sources of information that ProMED-mail receives on a daily basis. The first is subscriber input, most often firsthand reports or news stories from local or other outlets that subscribers forward to ProMED-mail. The second consists primarily of news information about emerging diseases outbreaks that ProMED-mail's staff and volunteer 'rapporteurs' identify through regular monitoring of electronic news media, other Listservs, and official and unofficial public health Web sites. All of this incoming information is communicated via the Internet, primarily through e-mail (Madoff 2004; Madoff & Woodall 2005).

Like other early warning outbreak systems, ProMED-mail faces the challenges of dealing with incoming reports that are unofficial and unverified. Because ProMED-mail posts its own reports directly to the public, it has developed an internal assessment process for vetting incoming information. On a given day a 'top moderator,' the ProMED-mail editor or one of the associate editors, acts as the focal point for all incoming and outgoing e-mail information. The top moderator makes an initial assessment of incoming e-mail reports and forwards those that are of relevance to a ProMED-mail subject area expert for further vetting, editing, and commentary. Vetted reports are copyedited, then returned to the top moderator for final review and dissemination through the ProMED-mail Website and one or more of its e-mail distribution lists (Madoff 2004).[37] ProMED-mail reports are also forwarded to WHO on a daily basis.

ProMED-mail has been recently characterized in terms that liken it to a global public health good. Madoff and Woodall (2005: 724) describe it as an initiative that has "developed and served the public health community." In their account, ProMED-mail's "goal was, and has always been, to serve global public health by acting as an early warning system for outbreaks of emerging diseases" (Madoff & Woodall 2005:724). There can be no doubt that ProMED-mail has made important contributions to global public health. Since its inception, it has spread global awareness of and helped mobilize early responses to EID outbreaks by identifying and reporting on them well in advance of formal notification to WHO.

ProMED-mail was established in a context of tension between the use of early warning outbreak detection systems to meet public health surveillance objectives and their use to meet national security and defense goals. At its inception ProMED-mail was far more closely aligned with bioweapons surveillance than its representation as a global public health good in EID control might suggest. The formal document announcing ProMED, a consensus statement produced following its inaugural meeting in 1993, represents ProMED as a response to the recommendations made by the CDC for heightened surveillance of microbial threats to U.S. national health (Morse et al. 1996). As outlined in the previous chapter, EID at this historical moment was a concept very much tied to U.S. national security interests and to the possibility of health threats stemming from the use of bioweapons. At the time it was written, the key authors of the ProMED statement all had close connections with the issue of biosecurity: Stephen Morse as a member of the Federation of American Scientists' Working Group on Biological and Toxin Weapons Verification, Barbara Hatch Rosenberg as coordinator of the Working Group, and Jack Woodall as a member of WHO's Gulf Task Force. All three authors were previously engaged in a debate about the use of international epidemiological surveillance to detect bioweapons and had argued strongly against the feasibility of establishing surveillance systems focused exclusively on bioweapons, while at the same time they had put forward the case for harmonizing early detection of natural and deliberate disease outbreaks (Morse 1992; Woodall 1992; Rosenberg 1992).

Our interview research confirms this history, pointing to how ProMED was initially established for explicit bioterrorism surveillance and was only later realigned to meet broader global public health goals in response to perceived funding constraints and internal pressures:

> [ProMED] wanted to set up, to get funding to set up a ring of institutions around the world which had the capability, rather like CDC has, of parachuting people into spots where there are suspicious outbreaks to find out whether they were due to bioterrorism or not . . . One important point about this was that we were set up, you see, to look for outbreaks that might be due to bioterrorism but, __ [name] convinced the Federation of American Scientists that they weren't going to get any money for bioterrorism watch at that time, but for any outbreaks we found and studied and reported on that were of interest to public around the world. (ProMED-mail Interview)

Of all WHO's unofficial sources of information on outbreak and other public health events, ProMED-mail has been the most written about, often by authors who are founders or editors of ProMED-mail. As suggested earlier, supporters of ProMED-mail are fond of arguing on behalf of the initiative by emphasizing its timeliness. ProMED-mail cofounder Jack Woodall and current ProMED-mail editor Lawrence Madoff have recently published a chronological discussion of ProMED-mail reports from 1994 to 2005 (Madoff & Woodall 2005). Their work demonstrates how news information and subscriber observations have been used to post reports of outbreaks on ProMED-mail, often weeks in advance of formal WHO announcements. Often quoted in arguments supporting and legitimating the initiative is a particularly favorite report, the February 10, 2003 ProMED-mail post from Stephen O. Cunnion that read "Have you heard of an epidemic in Guangzhou? An acquaintance of mine from a teachers' chat room lives there and reports that the hospitals there have been closed and people are dying." ProMED-mail enthusiasts claim the post as the first public report of the SARS outbreak released a full 2 weeks before the outbreak was announced by WHO (Madoff 2004: 227).

ProMED-mail and GPHIN are both early warning outbreak detection systems sourced in unofficial texts. They respond to the demand for faster detection of EID outbreaks and other threats to global public health, but they do so in quite different fashions. ProMED-mail operates through the communication capabilities of e-mail and seeks to continually expand its base of human subscribers and encourage amongst them norms of watchfulness and alert to local public health events that can be reported to ProMED-mail, vetted, and redistributed to the subscriber network. GPHIN, by contrast, innovates at the level of the electronic processes used to identify and retrieve relevant news reports from vast amounts of unstructured and undifferentiated Web-based information. GPHIN is a sophisticated intervention in the retrieval of Web-based news items for public health purposes. At its heart is filtering software that uses a custom-built taxonomy of keywords and Boolean search syntaxes to automatically scan news information for stories about potential infectious disease outbreaks and other threats to international public health. Those items are vetted and edited by GPHIN staff, then automatically translated and made available to GPHIN subscribers. In contrast to ProMED-mail, GPHIN does not rely on subscriber-based input, nor is the system public. The use of GPHIN is restricted to organizations with a demonstrated interest in the surveillance of public health emergencies, and fees vary according to such factors as organizational size and type (e.g., governmental versus nongovernmental) and the number of individual users (GPHIN Interview).[38]

We have concentrated on GPHIN and ProMED-mail given their historical importance at the turn of the 21st century for the establishment of global emergency vigilance. However, as we noted previously, there are many other event-based monitoring systems in existence, including MedISys (Health Threats Unit at Directorate General Health and Consumer Affairs of the European Commission 2007) and Argus, a U.S. government-funded system (Wilson, Polyak, Blake, & Collmann 2008). We find HealthMap of particular interest as it hybridizes the techniques of GPHIN and ProMED-mail. Launched in 2006, HealthMap is located at the Children's Hospital Informatics Program, Harvard Medical School, and seeks to "supplement existing public health systems by focusing on event-based monitoring of infectious diseases by leveraging Internet news and other electronic media" (Freifeld, Mandl, Ries, & Brownstein 2008: 151). Its main funder is Google Inc.[39] HealthMap uses Web-accessible information sources rather than the news aggregators upon which GPHIN relies (Brownstein et al. 2008: 1019).

It is similar to GPHIN in that it has a sophisticated automated scanning and translation capacity. Like ProMED-mail, but unlike GPHIN, HealthMap is available free of charge to anyone who wants to use it, including governments and travelers. ProMED-mail is one source for HealthMap's content, though it also uses news media, official alerts from WHO, and other designated Websites. The data are displayed on geographic maps (Freifeld et al. 2008: 154). One of HealthMap's current objectives is to go "beyond its role as an information provider to becoming an engaged, online community"[40] that operates similarly to Facebook or Twitter, a "social networking device" to link disease experts. Event-based monitoring is a growth area in contemporary public health, with competing systems trying to give the earliest alert of outbreak/emergency and an expanding repertoire of techniques.

B) Outbreak Verification

By harnessing the near real-time properties of Internet information exchange, GPHIN and ProMED-mail responded to the temporal requirements of a developing global emergency vigilance apparatus and its concern with outbreaks and other public health emergencies. GPHIN and ProMED-mail are significant public health innovations that offer a sophisticated technical architecture through which global health news was transformed into an important discursive resource for global health vigilance. However, from the standpoint of WHO and international infectious disease control more generally, the information sources of GPHIN and ProMED-mail presented a vexing challenge: They are unofficial accounts. Organizing a WHO-mediated system of global vigilance of significant global public health threats on the basis of news accounts and firsthand observations would be tantamount to releasing WHO international credibility to the vagaries of rumor. While GPHIN and ProMED-mail resolved the problem of timeliness by bypassing epidemiological case reports and relying on news and other sources of unofficial knowledge, using these sources presented the problem of securing the dependability and veracity of report. International public health officials responded to this problem by developing a system of outbreak verification.

As one of its founders recalls, GPHIN met with initial resistance from public health scientists on the question of unverified data:

> We went to the first CDC-sponsored international conference on emerging infectious diseases and we set up a little dinner with major countries: England, Italy, Germany, CDC representing United States, and a few others . . . And we basically presented the concept and, well, we were very enthusiastic and convinced it was going to work, and we were met with pure skeptics, like come on, this isn't traditional surveillance, because we weren't there to learn the details of how many

of each case. We just wanted to have rough ballpark figures of how many cases there were, like country Z has 40 cases of Y and 10 deaths. We didn't care so much if it was 42 or 39 . . . We weren't into the real detailed epi kind of data you know, that you need for real outbreak investigation, that kind of study. We just wanted to know if there was something going on. So we weren't that interested in precision; and of course most of the people in that meeting were classic epidemiologists, and they basically said "Ah, interesting" and walked away. (GPHIN Interview)

For those other than WHO (see succeeding text for discussion) attending the invitational dinner at the First International Conference on Emerging Infectious Diseases (1998), GPHIN was uninteresting and unintelligible as it did not conform to the existing schema for epidemiological surveillance.

Early warning outbreak detection engaged in a struggle for recognition with what has come to be called 'traditional' surveillance. It was and still is referred to as "monitoring" rather than surveillance (GPHIN Interview); 'monitoring' has the sense of intermittent/episodic measurement and 'surveillance' has the sense of continuous measurement.[41] Since its invention in the 1950s surveillance has, with certain exceptions (see the discussion of Alexander Langmuir earlier in this chapter), been based on units of information that have been medically/scientifically verified, and both GPHIN's data source and output (alerts) were considered unverified—mere rumor. But GPHIN and other online early warning outbreak detection systems created something that had not previously existed: a secondary analysis of rumor.

As we have already outlined earlier in this chapter, since the inception of WHO, its officials have on occasion used news reports to prompt inquiries to confirm or disconfirm outbreaks. But as an unofficial, unverified source of information about outbreak and other public health events, news had not been legally recognized and incorporated into WHO's notification system. Under the terms of the ISR (1951) and the IHR (1969), Member States had no obligation to respond to news accounts of outbreaks occurring within their territories, and WHO had no authority to publicly comment on outbreaks that had been reported through news.

The founders of GPHIN were well aware of the gap between a system of outbreak detection that relied on unofficial information and the legally mandated operation of the WHO-coordinated system of international notification regarding infectious disease outbreaks and other public health events. From the outset, it was clear that for GPHIN to be of relevance to WHO and the broader global public health community, its reports would need to be confirmed in some fashion. Equally clear was that GPHIN itself lacked the authority to provide the required form of verification:

You could not call the Minister of Thailand, or wherever, as the director of GPHIN and say "We've been getting these reports of outbreaks in Thailand." The Minister could turn and say, "Well, we have no re-sponsibility to do anything or to respond to your call in any particular way." (GPHIN Interview)

WHO representatives attending the 1998 International Conference on Emerging Infectious Diseases (discussed previously) suggested to the Health Canada officials that GPHIN alerts could be verified through WHO. WHO was the only organization that had the international diplomatic mandate to organizationally secure verification of unofficial outbreak reports by com-municating with country members through its regional and national WHO offices (GPHIN Interview). GPHIN thus established a partnership with WHO whereby GPHIN would supply unofficial outbreak information and WHO would verify the information through its official country contacts. That relationship was formalized in 2001, after some years of development, in an agreement between WHO and Health Canada, acting on behalf of GPHIN.

Both GPHIN's and ProMED-mail's alerts are sent to WHO for verifica-tion. WHO's outbreak verification system is organizationally located in WHO's Geneva-based Outbreak Alert and Response Operations Team, a component of the Global Outbreak Alert and Response Network (GOARN). Both GPHIN and ProMED-mail are GOARN partners. GOARN and the Outbreak Alert and Response Team fall under the responsibility of WHO's Epidemic and Pandemic Alert and Response Programme. The formation of GOARN began in 1997, and the network was formally launched in 2000 (Heymann & Rodier 2004). GOARN was established to deal with grow-ing global public health concerns about limitations in national infectious disease surveillance and response capacity and the economic and other con-sequences of delays in reporting and acting on outbreaks. GOARN is a voluntary network of over 110 institutions that pools human and technical resources to rapidly identify, confirm, and respond to outbreaks of inter-national importance. It is what one of the WHO interview participants termed "a set of managed relationships, relationships with institutions, not individuals" (WHO Interview). One of GOARN's key contributions to global emergency vigilance is the deployment of multidisciplinary response teams to assist local health authorities in the investigation and contain-ment of outbreaks and other public health events. Its practices include field investigations, confirmation of diagnosis, laboratory services, outbreak communications, and the provision of logistics including staff and supplies of therapeutics, vaccines, and laboratory equipment.[42]

To give some idea of the scale of operations for outbreak alert and response at WHO, including outbreak verification, we note that in an October 2006 interview, a WHO research participant reported the total biennial budget of Epidemic and Pandemic Alert and Response as US$220 million, but the effective budget allocated by WHO was US$11 million; that is, 5% of the biennial budget came from WHO's regular budget. The remainder of the budget was raised directly from donors. WHO research participants expressed frustration that much of their work time was spent raising US$2 million per week (WHO Interview). WHO supplies GOARN with a small administrative staff, including an operational support team, a project manager, and assistance for a steering committee (Hitchcock et al. 2007: 218). Although most members cover their own participation costs, there is no budget provided by WHO for GOARN work, and field responses must be funded by staff through fundraising outside WHO each time a response occurs (Chu 2005). The U.S.-based Nuclear Fund Initiative provided GOARN with a revolving fund of US$500,000, the WHO-NTI Global Emergency Response Fund, which may be allocated to immediate mobilization of response teams provided that the expenditures are later reimbursed (Hitchcock et al. 2007: 218). The governance infrastructure of global emergency vigilance does not have robust funding. WHO's outbreak alert and response programming is brilliance on a small budget.

Verification, as a practice that seeks to confirm or disconfirm the accuracy of an uncertain account or report, has historical precedents in international infectious disease surveillance. For example, in his writings on the global campaign to eradicate smallpox, Henderson (2007: 504–505; 1976) noted the routine practice of verifying suspected cases of smallpox detected through "secondary surveillance systems." To enhance primary surveillance networks that relied on reporting through the formal health care system, smallpox surveillance was typically extended to such groups as agricultural workers, block development officers, the police, security forces, school teachers, and students. Suspected cases reported by such informal sources were subject to routine investigation and verification by surveillance teams. From the mid-1970s in India, Pakistan, and Bangladesh "systematic house by house searches, the ultimate in the development of secondary surveillance systems" (Henderson 1976: 22) were conducted. In addition to these periodic special searches, smallpox cases were detected through the use of "specially organized searches in problem areas such as slum areas of cities and these, on occasion, were conducted not house by house but room by room" (Henderson 1976: 23). Beyond the level of local secondary surveillance, WHO from the late 1960s queried national governments to verify national reports and non-reports of smallpox cases (Henderson 1976: 27). What distinguishes WHO's outbreak verification and alert system from earlier practices of verification is the extent to which it has been propelled by news and how, as an organizational and technical innovation, it has fundamentally transformed the knowledge base of international infectious disease surveillance.

The operation of WHO's outbreak verification and alert system has been described in detail by Grein and colleagues. Grein et al. (2000: 97) refer to outbreak verification as "a new approach to global disease surveillance" the principal aim of which is to inform public health professionals "about confirmed and unconfirmed outbreaks of international public health importance". Outbreak verification can be thought of as a sequence of practices for the institutional processing of news and other unofficial reports of outbreak according to the formal relevancies of global emergency vigilance. It involves assessment and investigative work to select from amongst all incoming reports those that meet the criteria for a genuine outbreak/emergency of global public health concern. Outbreaks that do not meet the required criteria are archived over the course of the process, which at the end yields confirmed outbreaks. Outbreak verification is a process rich in textual flows of information that transforms unconfirmed rumor into officially confirmed outbreaks of global public health significance that can be publicly communicated as outbreak alerts. It creates conditions for public announcement of outbreaks while it also initiates WHO-mediated efforts to contain them.

WHO's outbreak alert and verification system was developed at the same time that WHO undertook a major revision of the IHR (1969). Grein and colleagues describe WHO's outbreak verification at a time prior to the completion of the revisions. The use of informal news accounts by WHO was authorized by a resolution adopted by the World Health Assembly prior to the completion of the revision of the IHR (2005).[43] As detailed in Chapter 4, the IHR revisions were in part driven by the forms of experimentation in notification and response to outbreaks developed by the Outbreak Verification Team and GOARN. The process Grein et al. described in 2000 was created with a view to harmonization with the planned revisions of the IHR (2005). During an interview conducted in 2006, members of the Outbreak Verification Team noted that the only significant change to the processes and circumstances described by Grein and colleagues in 2000 was an increase in the volume of incoming information and a shift in the relative proportion of official and unofficial reports in favor of the former.

The first step in outbreak verification is to determine whether reports are of potential international public health importance. The criteria used in that determination have been recently codified in the IHR (2005) as criteria for designating events that may constitute a public health emergency of international concern. They include such factors as the potential for the event to spread internationally, whether its public health impact may be considered serious, the degree to which it is unexpected, the potential need for international assistance, and the risk of interference with travel or trade. In an interview, a member of the Outbreak Alert and Response Operations Team described the multiple forms of judgment that are drawn upon to make preliminary assessments of news and other forms of unverified outbreak information.

LW/EM: But if it's unverified information, then how do you judge the quality?

Research Participant: That is very difficult at times, and therefore your judgment is based on the disease itself. So for example, diarrheal disease outbreaks are reported every day. There's an awful lot of noise and

there's small outbreaks, large outbreaks, you know, wedding party outbreaks all the way through to a massive cholera outbreak in a refugee
camp, whereas other signals associated with things like hemorrhagic
fevers are much more precise. For example, report of an outbreak of
hemorrhagic fever from London is geographically not as relevant as an
outbreak report of 16 cases of fever with bleeding in northern Gabon,
where we've seen four outbreaks in the last 5 years. So it would depend
on the history of that syndrome in the particular geographic context.
It'll depend on the nature of the investigation that's been carried out
thus far, what the source is and what the source is reporting, and it'll
also depend on our assessment of the strength of the health system in
that country. (WHO Interview)

The preceding passage emphasizes the contextual factors in making
assessments, drawing attention to considerations related to the nature
of the infection, its geographical context, and the country's capacity to
respond.

Issues related to the quality of the unofficial source were also cited as significant for making preliminary assessments. Interview participants noted
that the filtering activities of GPHIN were helpful in removing "irrelevant
reports." They also emphasized assessments of the quality of information
sources, privileging firsthand accounts from established nongovernmental
organizations (NGOs) and raising questions about the neutrality of news
reports:

If the report happens to be from an NGO field manager who has just
seen a thousand people die with symptoms remarkably like meningitis, then the veracity of that report has to be taken absolutely. You've
got to trust the source on the ground who is actually seeing it. You
would put a lot more energy into the follow-up on that than you
would on some opposition newspaper in Venezuela that reports that,
you know, the government is researching smallpox and there's been
an accident . . . You can get out-of-context reports . . . politically motivated reporting on hemorrhagic fever or smallpox in particular, and
there are people out there who know that. They throw red herrings
into the system, so you can get that sort of thing. But I think the
[GPHIN] analysts in Canada have helped because that first filtration
helps because a lot of the stuff that's hopefully irrelevant is pulled out
early. (WHO Interview)

Assessment judges which sources are reliable; it is in part an exercise in the
boundaries of social trust.

Reports that are judged to be of potential international public health
interest pass to verification, the second stage of the outbreak verification process. Those that do not pass to verification are archived. During

verification, information from the preliminary assessment of reported outbreaks is shared with contacts from WHO's Regional Offices. Those contacts seek "confirmation of details from health authorities in the countries concerned, usually through the WHO representative" (Grein et al 2000: 99). Information from unofficial sources working in the field, such as the International Red Cross, may also be sought out at this time (Grein et al. 2000). The end result of verification is a decision about whether the reported event is a true outbreak ("observed number of cases exceeds expected number of cases in a given population for a given period" [Grein et al. 2000: 99]) and the criteria related to international public health significance. In interviews, members of the Outbreak Alert and Response Operations Team emphasized that verification is rarely secured on the basis of a single source of information. By contrast, it was described as a process of triangulation that involves ongoing consultations with national health officials and a mixture of official and unofficial information that produces "an approximation of the truth."

The final stage of the outbreak verification process is dissemination. WHO currently communicates disease outbreak information in a variety of ways. First, the Outbreak Verification List is distributed weekly to over 800 subscribers. Subscribers include WHO and UN staff, national health departments, field epidemiology training programs, and NGOs (Grein et al. 2000). The Outbreak Verification List includes information on confirmed outbreaks as well as outbreaks still under investigation. For this reason, access is restricted to subscribers. Second, reports of confirmed outbreaks of international public health significance are published in the Disease Outbreak News on the WHO Web site. In 2008 such reports numbered from 1 to 16 per month (see http://www.who.int/csr/don/en/). Reports of outbreaks in the Disease Outbreak News often follow an established narrative based on case information. Typical information communicated includes the reporting national health ministry, the date or dates of report, the circumstances and history of the case, the methods of diagnosis used, and the measures taken in response to the outbreak or other public health emergency. Finally, extended analyses of confirmed outbreaks are reported in the *Weekly Epidemiological Record*, a bilingual (English/French), official WHO publication available online to the public.[44]

Our account of outbreak verification and of outbreak detection emphasizes how public health officials introduced innovations in the ways online news was drawn upon and responded to in the technical apparatus of international infectious disease surveillance. We note here, however, that our research participants repeatedly underscored that social science and other research interested in innovative information technology can obscure how outbreaks are contained by human response in the field:

> The reporting in the general media . . . and in the scientific press always goes to the sexy innovative technology being used to save the world . . .

But at the end of the day when I see people's lives saved it's because we have vaccine stockpiles, and it's because we can get things to the field, and it's because government out-workers stay at their posts and don't run away when they see a hemorrhagic fever case. So the success of epidemic containment to a point has been improved by our ability to detect signals. But the reality on the ground is that we still have to do very difficult and dangerous work in the field . . . and the partnerships needed to do that get under-recognized . . . Whereas those of us international adventurers who have brand new ideas about how the Internet is going to save the planet get the recognition and the visibility because all we have to do is say the right words and people want to come and talk to us . . . and sometimes I get annoyed because what we do here is overinterpreted as high tech when in fact it's about how do we use technology to support the real deal, which is trying to stop epidemics which really involves people. (WHO Interview)

While outbreak verification represents an organizational response to the nonveridical character of unofficial outbreak information, it also represents the point of entry into field response to contain outbreak and other public health emergencies. Our interview participants stressed that requests for verification made by WHO's Outbreak Alert and Response Operations Team are always accompanied by an offer of assistance. Requests for verification are the starting point for dialogue with national public health authorities about the scale and nature of potential support from GOARN to contain the outbreak. WHO research participants emphatically stated that WHO's contact of countries during the verification process should not be interpreted solely as a demand for transparency but rather as a service offer: a "means to engage the international community in assisting that country to contain the epidemic" through the offer of vaccines, medications and personnel at the time of the verification process (WHO Interview).

Relations between Official and Unofficial Knowledge

Thus far in this chapter we have documented the organizational presence of news in public health knowledge of outbreaks/emergencies during the postcolonial and global emergency vigilance periods. First we described how news during the postcolonial period was routinely drawn upon as a practical knowledge in the day-to-day work of WHO officials. Then, turning to global emergency vigilance, we explored the incorporation of online news as a fundamental discursive resource in contemporary early warning outbreak detection and alert. We now undertake a comparative analysis of the place of news in the two periods, giving particular attention to the changing boundary between official and unofficial ways of knowing about outbreaks/emergencies.

Although unofficial news information has been used for public health purposes in both the postcolonial and global vigilance periods, there are important differences between the two periods in how news entered public health knowledge. First, the methods through which news items have been identified and collected for public health purposes vary. Second, the two periods are characterized by fundamental dissimilarities in the social organization of the relation between news and public health. Third, the material form of news in the two periods is characterized by a shift from printed paper to digitized information flows. Fourth, the political and legal definitions of the relation between official report and unofficial news information are divergent. Fifth, the boundary between official and unofficial knowledge of outbreak and other public health events shifts from a relation of dominance to parity. Overall there is a movement from an occasional informal reliance on news in the postcolonial period to its systematic incorporation within a new system of knowledge relations in global emergency vigilance.

In the postcolonial period, news reports entered into international public health practice in an ad hoc way that drew on social practices found outside public health. News stories were identified by literate persons, some of whom were public health personnel, who read newspapers and magazines as part of their leisure practice rather than their work practice. Clipping and forwarding stories from printed newspapers and magazines was a conventional social practice on which public health drew as an informal method for acquiring news reports. The choice of the publications from which the news clippings came was not made on the basis of explicit public health criteria. During this period there were no attempts to systematically collect news reports of outbreak. For public health authorities, dealing with news reports about communicable disease outbreak was a practitioner knowledge that was learned on the job rather than being a formal part of public health training.

By contrast, early warning outbreak detection and alert introduces institutional processes for systematically gathering unofficial outbreak/event reports, contributing to a new organizational presence for news in international communication about outbreak. In the global emergency vigilance period, the collection and identification of unofficial outbreak/event reports became specialized and coordinated through new organizational sites such as GPHIN and ProMED-mail. News and other forms of unofficial information acquired an institutionally recognized source of public health knowledge subjected to systematic data collection. Online outbreak detection and alert shifts the reading of news to the site of global public health practice, introducing standardized electronic monitoring created on the basis of text-mining expertise and reasoning. Outbreak detection and alert has a reflexive relation to its data source that is subject to revision both in terms of sources sampled and in terms of its automated categories. That reflexivity relies on public health knowledge, linguistic expertise, and familiarity with news narratives in order to select search terms and word associations in multiple languages to form search strategies that might yield news reports of greatest public health relevance.

The social organization of the relation between news and public health in global emergency vigilance thus differs sharply from that of the postcolonial period. In emergency vigilance, news became formally incorporated into the work practices of online early warning outbreak detection and outbreak verification. But during the postcolonial period no public health units had a dedicated and systematic relation to news other than those that were charged with producing news releases about the activities of the public health organization itself.

The material form of the unofficial information sources drawn upon in the two periods also differs in important ways. Early warning outbreak detection presupposes the widespread publication of news in online form; its unofficial sources of information have a digitized form rather than a printed, paper form. Digitized news extends the scale of outbreak detection, opening it up to quantities of textual information that would have been inconceivable during the postcolonial period. The online character of news reports also permits outbreak detection to proceed in a temporally continuous rather than discontinuous fashion. In the postcolonial period unofficial news of outbreak was identified through the temporally discrete and discontinuous reading practices of individuals who were connected to an arbitrarily identified printed corpus. By contrast, early warning outbreak detection and alert is based on continuous monitoring 24 hours a day, 7 days a week of a reflexively chosen online corpus.

Postcolonial knowledge of outbreak and global emergency vigilance also fundamentally differ in how the distinction between official and unofficial knowledge is determined politically and legally. In the mid-1990s the political demand on WHO for speedy detection of EID outbreaks decisively broke with the mild country expectations about timely epidemiological communications that characterized the postcolonial period. The country members of WHO, led by the USA, pressured WHO to develop systems for EID surveillance that would give faster and more comprehensive knowledge of outbreaks than previous epidemiological communications. They demanded that WHO achieve not simply fast knowledge of known and actual diseases, but a public health knowledge adequate to the unknown and the potential in the microbial world. These demands were not only about digital fastness (the usual way that social scientists analyze global online communications), but also about the creation of a surveillance technique that could activate EID at the level of its meaning. The response to this problematizing of postcolonial communications was the development of early warning outbreak detection and alert as an expertise in the public health handling of unofficial outbreak information.

David Fidler, in the context of analyzing the actions of WHO during the SARS outbreak of 2003, argues that WHO's capacity to use unofficial surveillance information and issue global alerts about infectious disease outbreaks "changes the way in which states exercise their sovereignty" (Fidler 2004b: 144). He maintains that unofficial outbreak information and global alerts act as a "global health governance pincer that squeezes the state's sovereign decision of whether to report outbreak information and to cooperate with WHO and other countries" (ibid). We concur with Fidler that outbreak detection, sourced in unofficial information, has modified official practices of outbreak notification. As one GPHIN interviewee observed, "[i]nformation could come from any particular place at any time. And governments were no longer in control of their information" (GPHIN Interview).[45]

The systematic use by WHO of unofficial sources in outbreak detection systems occurred under the political authority of the World Health Assembly in a long series of resolutions (WHO 2005; Annex 1, Policy Context: 42–43). The legal confirmation of WHO's practices for gathering and announcing unofficial information—together with issuing travel advisories, global alerts, and other temporary recommendations during an international public health emergency—were authorized by the World Health Assembly in May 2003 only after these powers had been used during the SARS outbreak (Fidler 2004b: 143). Fidler emphatically underscores this point: "The widespread acquiescence of sovereign states to the aggregation of power by WHO in the absence of any express policy or legal framework is astonishing (Fidler 2004b: 143)." We note that Fidler is a lawyer, and lawyers are rarely astonished. WHO's use of unofficial information in outbreak detection also predated GOARN's formal launch in 2000, as one of our WHO research participants observed:

> Early on in the revision when we set up the Global Outbreak Alert and Response Network and we included GPHIN in that, there was a great concern by our legal department that we were taking information from sources other than countries, which is where we had a mandate under the International Health Regulations. We now have a mandate to take information under the IHR from other sources. (WHO Interview)

Legal issues of state sovereignty over outbreak information under the IHR (1969) were present as early as 1997 when outbreak verification began at WHO (Grein et al. 2000: 97).

The IHR (2005) gave legal authorization to the increasing importance of unofficial knowledge in global surveillance: "WHO may take into account reports from sources other than notifications or consultations" (IHR 2005: Art. 9). The public release of unofficial information is carefully specified. WHO is required to evaluate unofficial reports "according to established epidemiological principles" and contact the "State Party" to obtain verification (IHR 2005: Art. 9). The IHR (2005) outlines a detailed standard for verification, which requires the "State Party" to acknowledge requests for verification and respond to WHO with public health information within 24 hours of the initial request. For the first time in the history of the IHR, WHO is given legal authority to release information "to the public if other information about the same event has already become publicly available and there is a need for the dissemination of authoritative and independent information" (IHR 2005: Art. 11), providing that its country members have already received the information from WHO. This provision enables WHO to disseminate unofficial news of outbreak and other public health events, if necessary without the consent of the nation state(s) in which the outbreak or other public health emergency is occurring.

The IHR (2005) formulates a new legal relation between the official and unofficial knowledge of public health events. Whereas under the IHR (1969) only official knowledge was recognized and unofficial knowledge was not, the revised IHR (2005) recognize two sources of knowledge—the official and the unofficial; the recognition alters the relation between the two terms. The IHR (2005) give legal form to the increasing importance of unofficial knowledge in early warning outbreak detection and authorize WHO to use and publicly release reports other than those provided through country notification and consultation. This implicitly introduces a third term between official and unofficial knowledge that had not legally existed prior to 2003: unofficial knowledge of record. The term 'knowledge of record' is defined as a legally authorized statement that may be publicly announced. Prior to the formation of global emergency vigilance, only official knowledge of outbreak was a knowledge of record; unofficial knowledge could never become a knowledge of record. But under the IHR (2005) a third possibility exists: Unofficial knowledge can become a knowledge of record for WHO when a public health event, judged by WHO to be an international public health emergency, has received widespread publicity. The third term links knowledge of record, which was formerly possible only on the basis of official knowledge, with unofficial knowledge, which was formerly never a knowledge of record. The existence of the third term has a series of effects on the prior official–unofficial binary.

The IHR (2005) dismantle the legal conditions that had made the news strategy of shame against WHO so effective in previous decades. When WHO publicly announced the 1970 cholera epidemic in Guinea without prior official confirmation, it created a crisis among its membership as the precedent threatened the principle of sovereign control of epidemiological information. Yet widespread media coverage of the cholera outbreak preceded WHO's public confirmation of it. The changed legal status of unofficial knowledge in the IHR (2005) makes a recurrence of this situation impossible, as WHO is legally authorized to speak under similar conditions. The changed legal status of unofficial knowledge in the IHR (2005) enhances WHO against dangers to its symbolic capital from the ongoing news strategy of shame.

Online early warning outbreak detection has many effects on the boundary between the official and the unofficial. Early warning systems have made it difficult for countries to conceal outbreaks and other public health events, a practice based on the reasonable fear of damage to their economies or prestige. Realizing this, the country members of WHO increasingly officially report outbreaks. In an analysis of state responses to SARS and subsequent outbreaks, David Heymann has argued that a change has occurred in the international norms of public health reporting, characterized by "open and transparent collaboration among countries" (2006: 3) and "global solidarity in the detection and validation of" outbreak (2006: 4). Heymann (2006: 1) cites internal WHO statistics that indicate that from January 2001 to October 2004 only 39% of unverified (initial) outbreak reports to WHO were reported by ministries of health; the remaining 61% came from unofficial sources. In October 2006, WHO research participants estimated that roughly 50% of unverified reports received by WHO were from unofficial sources. WHO data for the period January 1, 1998 to December 31, 2005 indicate that the proportion of total verified events (N=1256) supplied by official, formal sources as opposed to GPHIN and other unofficial sources increased sharply in 2004 and 2005 after the SARS outbreak (Mawudeku et al. 2007: 311, Fig. 23.4). Yet, as one of our WHO research participants observed, GPHIN had not diminished in importance:

> It would be wrong to say it's [GPHIN's] less significant because countries are reporting because they know if they don't, GPHIN will. So I think it's not less significant. It's just that the norm is changing, and countries see it to their advantage to report . . . National systems are different than GPHIN. GPHIN is the safety net. (WHO Interview)

Sovereign states obviously did not disappear at the turn of the 21st century, but they are now reactive to the presence of a transnationalized system of outbreak communications that they themselves have politically and legally authorized. Early warning outbreak detection and alert creates a systematic, transnationalized, unofficial knowledge of outbreak and other public health events that is anticipated by sovereign states and that affects their official notification activities.

As a result of both early warning outbreak detection and the changed legal status of unofficial information in international infectious disease control, sovereign states became aware that online news reports may be picked up by international outbreak detection systems. The result has been attempts by sovereign states to control online news of communicable disease outbreaks in their jurisdictions. It is well known that the People's Republic of China has attempted to control online domestic news of outbreak ("China and the Internet" 2006). During the course of our research we were also informally told of similar practices found in the USA, where online news stories about domestic communicable disease outbreaks have been observed to disappear.

The sourcing of outbreak detection in online postings has created political struggles around the control of digitized news of outbreak. Online data are transnationalized and largely independent of sovereign control, but persons and corporate groups who post outbreak information on the Internet sometimes do so at risk to themselves. ProMED-mail confers annual Awards for Excellence in Outbreak Reporting on the Internet, many of which go to individuals whose actions have placed them at risk of prosecution and coercive practices. In 1998 ProMED-mail gave one of its annual awards to Dr. Tan Poh Tim, a pediatrician in Sarawak, Malaysia, who released information about an enterovirus outbreak that had killed at least 50 children there in 1997.[46] When Taiwanese officials issued an appeal on the Internet in 1998 for information about diagnosis and treatment related to an outbreak among children, Dr. Tan Poh Tin posted information on ProMED-mail related to cases that she had personally dealt with the year prior, information that had not yet been officially released by Malaysia. In an interview, a ProMED-mail official noted to us that Dr. Tan was threatened with imprisonment by the Malaysian government and that the chancellor of her university had faced pressure to fire her.

During the postcolonial period, official communications were dominant over unofficial. Epidemiological information about outbreaks was conventionally represented in public health texts as a pyramid of report based on officially reported cases. But in the period of global emergency vigilance, knowledge of outbreak and other public health events is represented as having two parallel channels in a relation of parity: case-based surveillance and event-based monitoring. The enhanced utility and status of unofficial knowledge in online outbreak detection systems is present in the schematic drawings of epidemiological information in the publications of WHO and WHO officials. *Asia Pacific Strategy for Emerging Diseases* contains a figure that represents early warning systems with two main surveillance types: case based and event based (WHO 2005: 27, Fig. 1). Case-based surveillance uses official sources, and event-based surveillance uses unofficial ones. Together they generate a signal for assessment. A similar representation of contemporary epidemiological information occurs in an article written by members of the Department of Communicable Disease Surveillance and Response, Alert and Response Office at WHO headquarters in Geneva (Formenty et al. 2006: 12, Fig. 2). In this figure, titled "Warning Procedures and Response to Epidemics," epidemiological information of outbreak is represented with two inputs labeled "formal" and "informal," which again appear at the same level.

Unofficial knowledge of outbreak is now reflexively known to public health officials as a valuable source of knowledge rather than dismissed as irrelevant rumor. Global public health security is now routinely conceptualized to involve a combination of official and unofficial sources, case-based and event-based information. For example, in an analysis of disease surveillance in Europe, Paquet and colleagues (2006) use the term "epidemic intelligence" to refer to both official and unofficial sources of knowledge. Epidemic intelligence refers to "all activities related to early identification of potential health hazards, their verification, assessment and investigation in order to recommend public health control measures" (Paquet et al. 2006: n.p.). This rendering of intelligence repeats uses of the term "epidemiological intelligence" found in the first half of the 20th century (Bashford 2004: 134). Epidemic intelligence coordinates within a single concept both case-based data from established epidemiological surveillance systems *and* event-based data from unofficial sources.

Postcolonial epidemiological communications were characterized not only by the division between official and unofficial communications, but also by the dominance of the official over the unofficial. In the period of global emergency vigilance, official and unofficial communications are conceptualized as having equal status, an increase in the status of unofficial communications. The result for epidemiological communications was a yoking together of official pyramid and unofficial flat plane in a relation of parity.

Conclusion

The popularization of the EID concept in global public health circles challenged established approaches to international communicable disease surveillance at WHO. The prospect of constant microbial mutability and the emergence of previously unknown diseases as potential threats to global public health impelled new demands for faster and more extensive knowledge of global outbreaks. The very speed of unofficial outbreak reports, sourced largely in news media that had formerly shamed WHO internationally during the outbreak of pneumonic plague in Surat, India, during the mid-1990s, was turned into a resource for global public health.

In this chapter we have explored the changes to the technical apparatus of international communicable disease occasioned by EID. We have emphasized shifts in the knowledge relations of infectious disease surveillance, in particular, the relation between unofficial and official outbreak communication before and after the late 1990s. Our analysis treats news as an active form of knowledge that both propels and shapes organizational responses to the surveillance challenges posed by EID. Although news has been a part of international communicable disease control at WHO since it was formed, early warning outbreak detection alters the organizational status of news and its relationship to official knowledge of outbreak. Whereas prior to the late 1990s news had low status in a surveillance system that was dominated by official sources, the formal incorporation of news in early warning outbreak detection and alert systems elevated the status and utility of news within global disease surveillance.

We have argued that at the turn of the 21st century international communicable disease control was reconstructed as an emergency vigilance apparatus that is dedicated to identification of hazardous events. Early warning outbreak detection facilitates the time and space relations required for global emergency vigilance. It enables international public health authorities to identify outbreaks and other public health events when they were taking place and thus to make possible responses that contain outbreaks and other public health emergencies. The time of local outbreak and the time of international public health knowledge are made part of a single, continuous, accelerated global time. With respect to spatial relations, early warning outbreak detection uses transnationalized data. As a technique of global emergency vigilance, early warning outbreak detection and alert is a methodology that takes transnationalized, unofficial data and subjects it to systematic analysis, which makes possible a knowledge of outbreak that is substantively beyond sovereign power.

The shift in the knowledge base of international communicable disease control—later called 'global public health security'—represented by the new place of news in early warning outbreak detection was more than a technical accomplishment. It required transformations in the international legal framework governing WHO's infectious disease surveillance system. In this chapter we have touched on the agreements that were required to authorize the use of unofficial sources of outbreak information by WHO, including revisions to the IHR (1969). In the next chapter we turn our attention to the revision process and the introduction of new public health concepts at international law that formally established a global emergency vigilance apparatus.

4 From Infectious Disease to Public Health Emergency

The previous chapter focused on news as an unofficial source of information for WHO about outbreaks and other public health events. It compared the relations between official and unofficial knowledge of outbreak before and after the invention of early warning outbreak detection. The present chapter centers on official knowledge of outbreak and other public health events, specifically how the IHR (1969) and the IHR (2005) conceptualize what it is that must be reported to WHO by its sovereign Member States.

The IHR (2005) define the primary current international health law dealing with infectious disease control across national borders. They are part of a long history of efforts dating to the mid-19th century to establish international legal frameworks that respond to the challenges presented by the international mobility of infectious diseases. Like earlier international legal instruments, the IHR (2005) express a tension between public health goals focused on minimizing the spread of international public health emergencies that include, but are not limited to, infectious diseases and economic goals focused on preserving international travel and trade. This tension is found in the central objective of the IHR (2005): "to prevent, protect against, control and provide a public health response to the international spread of disease in ways that are commensurate with and restricted to public health risks, and which avoid unnecessary interference with international traffic and trade" (IHR 2005: Foreword). The Regulations, like earlier instruments, outline two main requirements of States Parties.[1] The first relates to notification and addresses questions regarding what States Parties are required to report, to whom, and under what conditions. The second relates to protective measures that States Parties can take, primarily with respect to international trade and tourism, in response to outbreaks and other public health events occurring beyond their national borders.

The International Sanitary Conferences held in Europe during the second half of the 19th century failed to reach an agreement on sanitary measures to prevent the spread of infectious diseases until the First International Sanitary Convention went into force in 1892. Before and after 1892, the various iterations of international legal mechanisms for infectious disease control were subject to widespread discussion, debate, rethinking, and revision amongst public health officials, infectious disease specialists, and legal scholars (Dorolle 1968; Howard-Jones 1975; Goodman 1971; Fidler 1999, 2004b; Loughlin & Berridge 2002; Gostin 2004a). The most recent revision that transformed the IHR (1969) into the IHR (2005) was a matter of widespread global public health interest. The scale of revision undertaken was unprecedented in the history of international infectious disease surveillance, which caused leading commentators to refer to it as "an historic development for international law and public health" (Fidler & Gostin 2006: 85).

In this chapter we do not provide a full account of the revision process. Nor do we offer an exhaustive analysis of the many changes made to the revised Regulations; that work has been done by others (Fidler 2004a; Nicoll, Jones, Aavitsland, & Giesecke 2005; Merianos & Peiris 2005; Schatz 2005; Fidler & Gostin 2006). Instead, we offer an analysis of conceptual innovation in the notification requirements of the IHR (2005). Our analysis focuses on the concepts that define mandatory reporting requirements: what the sovereign states that are members of WHO must report to WHO about what is occurring in their own territories.

The IHR (1969) and the IHR (2005) construct the object of mandatory public health reporting quite differently. In the IHR (1969), WHO country members are required to report all local cases of four diseases that are named in a list: cholera, plague, smallpox, and yellow fever. The infectious disease list has been a consistent feature of legal language in international public health law since 1892. By contrast, the IHR (2005) require States Parties to report "events which may constitute a public health emergency of international concern" that occur within their territories (IHR 2005: Art. 6). It is the displacement of the infectious disease list by the concept of "events which may be considered a public health emergency of international concern" that we wish to better understand here. Mandatory reporting is reconstructed as notification of events rather than cases, as previously, and events are related to public health emergencies rather than infectious diseases. A double displacement has been effected: the unit of report and its target. We argue that the EID concept problematized the place of the infectious disease list in international health law by making emerging and potential infectious diseases salient for international public health governance. The disease list was also problematized in relation to bioweapons use.

We begin our comparative analysis of how mandatory reporting requirements are conceptualized in the IHR (1969) and the IHR (2005) by examining the infectious disease list in the IHR (1969) and its antecedents in international public health law. We then turn to the challenge the EID concept presented to the IHR (1969), describing the new legal concepts of the IHR (2005) that were developed to deal with the identification of new, emerging, and potential infectious diseases. We conclude with a comparative analysis of the forms of public health reasoning projected by the the concept of the public health event as opposed to the disease list, exploring how the coupling of algorithmic reasoning and qualitative risk assessment in the identification of events orient to the requirements of global emergency vigilance in a way that no list, however long, would ever be capable of doing.

The International Health Regulations (1969): A Disease List and its Critique

The IHR (2005) are the most important recent example of a form of international health cooperation that arose amongst European states in the 19th century, the organizational form of which privileges international agreement on formalized rules and procedures for controlling the cross-border spread of infectious disease. The formative moment in this system of cooperation was the International Sanitary Conference of 1851 held in Paris, in response to political and economic concerns about the failure of established quarantine measures to control cholera epidemics that spread across Europe between 1830 and 1847 (Howard-Jones 1975). It was not until 1892 that the first international treaty on infectious disease control went into effect.

From 1892 to 2005, international public health legislation conceptualized mandatory reporting requirements through lists of named diseases. The diseases—variously called "notifiable," "pestilential," or "quarantinable"—comprised a subset of infectious diseases that were in part selected in response to anxieties about "diseases of the East" coming into Europe and the USA, but also in relation to the protection of international traffic. A history that attends to the inscription of certain diseases within international public health law and the noninscription of others has yet to be written, other than for cholera (Bynum 1993b; Huber 2006). Our limited focus here is on the disease list itself as an enduring legal statement for defining mandatory reporting requirements in international public health law.

Under the Constitution of the World Health Organization, the World Health Assembly (the legislative body of WHO) is mandated to create and adopt regulations regarding "sanitary and quarantine requirements and other procedures designed to prevent the international spread of disease" (WHO 1948: Art. 21). In 1951, shortly after it was formed, WHO combined the roughly 13 international agreements regarding quarantine and sanitary measures then in effect into a "single set of international legal rules on infectious disease control" called the International Sanitary Regulations (ISR; see Hardiman 2003; Fidler 2001: 843). The ISR (1951) were an international agreement that applied to six named "quarantinable" diseases that were defined in the ISR as follows: "*'quarantinable diseases'* means plague, cholera, yellow fever, smallpox, typhus, and relapsing fever" (ISR 1951: Art. 1; italics in original). The "quarantinable diseases" in the ISR (1951) were thus defined by a list of named examples rather than analytically. They were known diseases that could be clinically diagnosed, that is, by signs and symptoms on examination and by laboratory confirmation, where locally or regionally available. Under the ISR (1951), quarantinable diseases were made "notifiable" to WHO: "Each health administration shall notify the Organization by telegram within twenty-four hours of its being informed that a local area has become an infected local area" (ISR 1951: Art. 3.1). Notifications (except for rodent plague) were to be followed by supplementary information about "the source and type of the disease, the number of cases and deaths, the conditions affecting the spread of the disease, and the prophylactic measures taken" (ISR 1951: Art. 4).

A major revision of the ISR (1951) occurred in 1969, a point at which they were renamed the International Health Regulations (IHR 1969; see Hardiman 2003). The IHR (1969) continued the practice found in the ISR (1951) of defining the object of notification through exemplification: "'diseases subject to the Regulations' (quarantinable diseases) means cholera, including cholera due to the El Tor vibrio, plague, smallpox, including variola minor (alastrim), and yellow fever" (IHR 1969: Art. 1). In 1981 the IHR (1969) were further revised to exclude smallpox in view of its eradication (Gostin 2004b).

The lists of quarantinable diseases in the ISR (1951) and in the IHR (1969) had been preceded since the last decade of the 19th century by a series of international legal agreements concerned with controlling the spread of infectious diseases across national boundaries. Like the ISR (1951) these international agreements did not apply to all infectious diseases known at the time, only to specific ones that were named in legislation. The International Sanitary Convention of 1892 named only cholera as subject to preventive measures.[2] The International Sanitary Convention of 1897 was restricted to plague (Abdullah 2007: 10).[3] By 1912 the list of quarantinable diseases in international health law had expanded to plague, cholera, and yellow fever: "Chaque Gouvernement doit notifier immédiatement aux autres Gouvernements le premier cas avéré de peste, de choléra ou de fièvre jaune constaté sur son territoire."[4] [Each government must immediately notify other governments about the first confirmed case of plague, cholera, or yellow fever ascertained in its territory.]

As a statement that appeared in the context of international public health law, the quarantinable disease list linked named diseases to many legal obligations, although the list as such was not an explicit public health concept. The IHR (1969) sought to coordinate international control of cross-border infectious diseases by specifying two main types of requirements for the sovereign states that were WHO members. The first requirement aimed to shape international communication about infectious disease between WHO and its Member States. The IHR (1969) specified that a Member State was required to notify WHO "within twenty-four hours of its being informed that the first case of a disease subject to the Regulations, that is neither an imported case nor a transferred case, has occurred in its territory" (IHR 1969: Art. 3). The disease list thus promoted a practice of notification based on recognizing local cases of abstract disease categories and reporting all cases within 24 hours. The second requirement related to responses on the part of sovereign members to infectious disease threats occurring outside their territories. Here the Regulations sought to temper protective acts on the part of neighbors and trading partners of countries that had reported cases of cholera, yellow fever, plague, or smallpox. They did so by specifying the maximum measures WHO country members could undertake to prevent the entry of infectious disease through incoming international trade and tourism.

The disease list was also fundamental to the conceptualization of the maximum health measures permitted under the IHR (1969). Part V of the 1981 revised version of the Regulations expressed maximum measures in terms of actions sovereign members could take with respect to human travelers, ships, aircraft, international cargo, baggage, and mail during different stages of an international voyage, that is, on departure, between departure and arrival, and on arrival. These actions were further defined by disease type. Thus, surveillance and isolation measures were specified for passengers who had been on board a vessel where cholera had been discovered, and criteria were outlined for identifying vessels that were to be regarded as infected with plague and so on. Through such measures the Regulations built a surveillance regime that projected into the field disease-specific forms of protective action.

While the disease list had a formative discursive presence throughout all versions of the IHR (1969), public health officials at WHO had little confidence in it. They also doubted the general effectiveness of the IHR (1969). In the period immediately following the enactment of the IHR (1969), WHO officials and others launched a strong critique of the IHR (1969). Many of the criticisms they developed were repeated in later critiques of the IHR (1969) in the mid-1990s after the invention of EID. The early critics structured their objections to the IHR (1969) in terms of a general critique of their timeliness. To support their critique of the Regulations as anachronistic and out of date, they objected to the limitations of the disease list, the challenges that growing international travel and trade posed for the IHR (1969), and the failure of Member States to comply with the notification requirements and maximum protective measures outlined in the Regulations.

WHO officials found great fault with the narrow focus of the IHR (1969) on cholera, plague, yellow fever, and smallpox. They argued that the restriction of the IHR's notification requirements to these four diseases demonstrated the Regulations' misstep with current public health priorities. For example, Boris Velimirovic of the Pan American Sanitary Bureau remarked that a number of infectious diseases significant from the standpoint of international travel at the time, such as tuberculosis, hepatitis, malaria, and meningitis, were not covered by the IHR (1969) (Velimirovic 1976). Others further noted that rather than addressing those diseases of greatest current significance, the IHR (1969) were focused on past diseases. With a rhetorical flourish characteristic of his writing, Eric Roelsgaard (Chief of Epidemiological Surveillance of Communicable Diseases at WHO) referred to cholera, plague, smallpox, and yellow fever as "pestilential diseases of the past" and argued that the IHR (1969) privileged them in matters of international traffic for largely historical reasons (Roelsgaard 1974: 267).

Increases in the scale and pace of international traffic offered a second basis of critique of the IHR (1969). Pierre Dorolle, then-Deputy Director-General of WHO, contrasted the speed and volume of international traffic at the time when the International Sanitary Regulations were adopted with those current around the time of his writing in 1968. He noted that from 1951 to 1967, the number of international airline passengers had increased over seven times from 7 million to 51 million per year. Meanwhile, the speed of air travel had quadrupled, while the number of passengers per aircraft had increased tenfold (Dorolle 1968). Writing 5 years later, Eric Roelsgaard (1974: 265) remarked on the growing phenomenon of world travel, stating "it is not unusual for the number of foreign visitors to a country during a year to exceed the number of inhabitants." The early WHO critics of the Regulations used the heightened pace of world traffic to call into question the speed of the surveillance provisions found in the IHR (1969). Dorolle, in particular, was concerned that the international movement of infection outpaced then-available mechanisms for international notification and distribution of information about disease outbreaks. At a broader level, the phenomenon of dramatically expanded world traffic raised the stakes for the IHR (1969), gesturing to a growing sphere of economic activity that they were meant to preserve.

In the years between 1969 and 1974, WHO officials also argued that the IHR (1969) had in practice failed to secure the notification requirements and countermeasures that were mandated to stop the international transmission of infectious diseases. On matters of notification, WHO critics observed a widespread and deep problem of noncompliance. Velimirovic, for example, noted that "a number of countries simply do not report at all. Some report only a small percentage of the cases or report them long after they have happened" (Velimirovic 1976: 479). In his assessment of how the Regulations functioned in practice, Pierre Dorolle remarked that during "normal" periods reports were received by WHO from countries that regularly experienced one of the four diseases subject to notification. However, "when a severe outbreak of a disease occur[red] in a new area the system of notifications [broke] down far too often" (Dorolle 1968: 789). Velimirovic and Dorolle provided a number of explanations about why countries underreported or failed to report infectious diseases under the terms of the IHR. Velimirovic noted that the surveillance capacities of countries characterized by poverty were not well developed, which created technical problems with the obligation to notify. Dorolle added that in some instances health authorities were simply unfamiliar with the disease, which substantially delayed reporting. However, the most common explanation offered by the critics relates to a second failure of the IHR (1969)—their inability to constrain or limit the protective measures taken by countries in response to outbreaks occurring beyond their national borders.

Among such measures in excess of those permitted by the IHR (1969) were significant disruptions to travel and tourism. For example, in response to earlier cholera outbreaks, many countries closed their borders and stopped the arrival of ships and airplanes from international destinations (Roelsgaard 1974). Some countries required that mail and other printed matter from countries reporting cholera be disinfected. One country "prohibited the import of tinned fruit" (Dorolle 1968: 790). Such actions were partly understood by WHO personnel in terms of the vulnerability of the Regulations to politics, particularly to country member concerns about appearing indecisive in the face of public demands for action in response to infectious disease epidemics. These actions were also explained by the absence of enforcement mechanisms within the IHR (1969), by the complexity of their rules, and by built-in loopholes that formally permitted WHO country members to supersede maximum measures during conditions of "grave danger to public health," a concept that was never fully defined (Velimirovic 1976: 479).

While the image of countries rushing to ban tinned goods provides a droll gloss to international responses to infectious diseases, the message of the early critics was a serious one. Countries failed to report outbreaks because of the often devastating economic hardships that followed when they did. The IHR (1969) had produced a system of surveillance in which noncompliance with maximum protective health measures directly fed into widespread failure to notify. The dismal extent to which the Regulations had met their stated objectives led the early critics to dismiss them as hopelessly dated. In their writings they drew on life cycle metaphors to refer to the IHR (1969) as "dead," and something that should be left to a "quiet withering away" (Velilmirovic 1976: 481). In a particularly vivid account, Velimirovic represented the ISR (1951) and the IHR (1969) as thoroughly anachronistic texts, "each revision [of which] was obsolete on the very day when it was published" (1976: 478). So deep was the early public health rejection of the IHR (1969) that critics did not express a general call for revising them. While some argued for changes to the IHR (1969), their strongest message was to respond to then-current problems in international disease control by closing the gap between North and South. In the words of Dorolle (1968: 792): "the only way of preventing the old plagues, and some new ones, from spreading from continent to continent and from country to country is to help the poorest nations of the world to reach such a level of economic and technical development that it will be possible for them to combat the evil at its source."

The critique of the IHR (1969) launched by WHO officials in the 1970s did not generate a compelling call to revise them, but important programme initiatives in the area of international infectious disease control nonetheless occurred. We briefly document the establishment of one such programme here, Emergency Aid in Epidemics, in order to evidence WHO practices around emergency response, the realities of international epidemiological communications about infectious disease outbreaks, and the ongoing patient frustration of WHO personnel with both these practices. Our comments here are based on archival research and display an internal critique situated in work practices, as distinguished from the critiques found in the published articles by WHO officials that we have just examined.

Aid during "emergencies" "upon the request or acceptance of Governments" had been made one of WHO's functions in its 1946 Constitution (WHO 1946: Art. 2). During the 1960s the standard WHO response to a country request for emergency aid was to send a consultant to do a field investigation. There were often considerable delays before a consultant reached the field. In 1966 the Scientific Group on Virus Diseases (WHO headquarters, Geneva) proposed a plan that would expedite WHO responses to requests for aid in emergency situations. Dr. W. Chas. Cockburn, who was Chief Medical Officer of Virus Diseases at WHO headquarters during the late 1960s and early 1970s, had the lead on this initiative. The resulting programme, Emergency Aid in Epidemics, was established in the same year the World Health Assembly gave approval to the IHR (1969).

The intent in setting up Emergency Aid in Epidemics was to create the possibility of obtaining rapid information about the causes of outbreaks, their extent, and their possible spread in order to develop control measures. From the experience of the Scientific Group on Virus Diseases, one of their biggest difficulties was to get information quickly concerning the etiology of a disease, its extent, what facilities were locally available, and what else was required.[5] Emergency Aid in Epidemics included panels of consultants who agreed to conduct field investigations on short notice in emergency situations. The purpose of developing panels of expert consultants was to expedite the process of getting consultants into the field. The programme stockpiled emergency supplies at WHO headquarters and its regional offices.[6]

In an internal critique of WHO practice, Dr. Cockburn showed that it had taken a consultant 7 months to reach the field in 1967/1968 after the Republic of Guinea had made a request for assistance to deal with a polio outbreak. Cockburn's memorandum provided a critique of WHO's response to the outbreak in one devastating table that detailed the chronology of the emergency assistance given to Guinea (see Table 4.1, p. 116–117). Cockburn noted that when the WHO consultant arrived in Guinea, "he found that 5–6 months earlier there had been an outbreak of over 200 paralytic cases."[7] But WHO had requested—fruitlessly—epidemiological data about the polio outbreak three times during July 1967. The first objective of Emergency Aid in Epidemics consisted precisely of "getting an expert to the

Table 4.1   Outbreak of Poliomyelitis in Guinea, Chronology of Events

Date	Event
16 June 1967	On request from AFRO[1], SUP[2] and VIR[3] arrange to send 50,000 doses vaccine free from the emergency supply
19 June 1967	VIR cable AFRO asking for information about outbreak and suggest they invite Institut Pasteur, Dakar to send consultant to collect specimens and assess situation
21 June 1967	Vaccine dispatched
23 June 1967	AFRO cable that suggestion for consultant impracticable because government has not made a request
4 July 1967	AFRO cable request for further doses but say no epidemiological information yet received from Guinea
6 July 1967	Arrangements made for dispatch of further 50,000 doses; AFRO again asked for epidemiological data and consultant from Dakar or Lyon proposed
10 July 1967	AFRO again ask Guinea for epidemiological data and now offer services of a consultant.
25 July 1967	AFRO cable Institut Pasteur, Dakar for consultant
3 August 1967	AFRO cable Guinea offering Dr. Barne, Institut Pasteur, Dakar for ten-day consultantship
25 August 1967	AFRO again cable Guinea asking for reply to their offer
31 August 1967	Guinea refuse to accept staff member from Institut Pasteur, Dakar
1 September 1967	AFRO cable VIR for names of other consultants
1 September 1967	VIR asks if Romanian is acceptable
13 September 1967	AFRO says yes
14 September 1967	VIR writes to Professor N. Cajal, Director, Institute of Inframicrobiology, Bucarest to ascertain if available
25 September 1967	Cajal cables VIR – will accept consultantship
25 September 1967	VIR cables AFRO

continued

continued

26 September 1967	AFRO cables Guinea
11 October 1967	AFRO reminds Guinea of offer of 26 September – requests reply
(about end of October)	Guinea agrees
1 November 1967	VIR and PERS[4] commence recruitment formalities
6 November 1967	DG cables Government of Romania for release of Cajal
29 November 1967	No reply from Government of Romania. I find on arrival for visit of Bucarest authority granted and Cajal can leave for Guinea beginning of January
14 December 1967	AFRO cable Guinea asking for agreement for Dr Cajal's visit
19 December 1967	Afro send reminder to Guinea
19 January 1968	Cajal arrives Brazzavile and proceeds to Guinea a few days later.

Notes 1. AFRO: WHO Regional Office for Africa 2. SUP: Supply Services, WHO 3. VIR: Virus Diseases, WHO, Geneva 4. PERS: Divisions of Personnel

Comment: This chronology of a polio outbreak in Guinea during 1967/1968 was used to illustrate the need for prompter emergency aid in epidemics. It shows that the WHO Regional Office for Africa and WHO headquarters had knowledge of the epidemic prior to being officially informed of it by the Republic of Guinea. The chronology also demonstrates the weak articulation between international public health knowledge of an outbreak and national knowledge of it.

Source: Outbreak of Poliomyelitis in Guinea, Chronology of Events in Appendix to Memorandum of Dr. W. Chas. Cockburn, Chief, VIR, to Dr, Payne, ADG, 4 March 1968, Subject: Emergency Aid for Epidemics of Virus Diseases. WHO Archives, WHO 10, Records of the Central Registry, WHO Headquarters: Sub-fonds 3 1955–1984, Emergency Aid in Epidemics, C8/180/2. Reproduced with permission of the World Health Organization.

field with all possible speed,"[8] intended as a corrective to the chronology of emergency aid found in the 1967/1968 polio outbreak in Guinea.

Polio was not part of the disease lists in the ISR (1951) and IHR (1969), but plague was. Despite the notification requirements of the ISR (1951), delays in emergency aid similar to the polio outbreak in Guinea occurred during a plague outbreak in the Democratic Republic of the Congo during 1968/1969. In January 1968, Dr. O. Tshiamu, Minister of Public Health of the Democratic Republic of the Congo, informed the WHO Regional Office for Africa about a plague outbreak and requested WHO help. With assistance from WHO headquarters, one consultant arrived in the Congo on March 24, 1969. The field response followed a protest to Dr. K. Raška, Director of the Division of Communicable Diseases at WHO headquarters, by Dr. S. Malafatopoulos, Director of Health Services for the WHO Regional Office for Africa, in a letter dated February 14, 1969: ". . . it is regretted that the WHO assistance to the Democratic Republic of the Congo, which was originally requested in January 1968, has not so far been implemented, in spite of voluminous correspondence."[9] Summarizing the historical experience of WHO in managing epidemics, a 1981 WHO report observed that "[a] delay of several weeks frequently occurs between the onset of an epidemic and the time it is declared and WHO's cooperation sought. Increasing mortality was frequently the earliest indicator to raise the alarm, particularly when epidemiological surveillance is deficient."[10] As we have shown, international public health officials had a limited official knowledge of outbreak partly because national health administrations sometimes did not know about outbreaks in their jurisdictions (see Table 4.1, Comment) and because they hesitated to report for fear of damage to their trade relations with other countries. Outbreak and epidemic occurred in local time and place, were weakly articulated to both official and unofficial knowledge in the first weeks of onset, and were incorporated in national and global time and space after the fact.

We have shown that the disease list defined the mandatory object of public health action in international health law related to infectious diseases between 1892 and the IHR (1969). We have also demonstrated that WHO personnel in the period leading up to and after the passage of the IHR (1969) had little confidence in the disease list and its associated practices of notification and protective measures. While the Regulations set the terms of international disease surveillance by specifying notification and protective measures requirements, they failed dismally at the level of application. Rather than actively shaping responses to infectious disease outbreaks, the Regulations were routinely ignored or bypassed. Yet simultaneously, WHO used its own internal critique of its actions in infectious disease control to create new programme initiatives, as we have briefly sketched in our discussion of Emergency Aid in Epidemics.

Yet, despite the disillusion with the place of the disease list in international public health, and despite the ability of WHO to engage in ongoing internal critique and organizational change, the disease list remained uncontested by any alternative concept of mandatory reporting requirements within international health law. The situation changed in the mid-1990s with the invention of the EID concept and its political backing by the global North.

Problematizing the Infectious Disease List

The year 1995 marked the beginning of the end of the disease list in international health law as the EID concept, formulated in terms of disease emergence and microbial potential for rapid genetic and ecological change, rendered obsolete its presupposition of fixed disease entities. However, we do not argue that the EID concept appears in the legal language of the IHR (2005). Instead, we maintain that the revision of the IHR (1969) was formulated, in part, as a response to EID. The legal language of the IHR (2005) addresses the political pressures on WHO to deal with EID by formulating legal concepts that are capable of encompassing the unknown, the uncertain, and the potential in infectious disease control, rather than only named diseases that have known causes and that can be diagnosed with certainty.

As we argued in Chapter 2, the EID concept was a central motivator of the revision of the IHR (1969). During the time the 48th World Health Assembly was convening (May 1–12, 1995), the first rapid-response WHO field team reached Kikwit in the Democratic Republic of the Congo to assist in public health measures to contain an outbreak of Ebola hemorrhagic fever. At the same time as the response team was beginning its work in Kikwit, the World Health Assembly passed Resolution 48.7, *Revision and updating of the International Health Regulations,* which referred to itself as "WHO's initiative on new, emerging and re-emerging infectious diseases" (World Health Assembly 1995a). Resolution 48.7 formulated communicable diseases in ecological and molecular genetic terms, which rendered the disease list in the IHR (1969) conceptually obsolete by using the scientific reasoning about EID found in the IOM's *Emerging Infections* (IOM 1992). In that same 48th World Health Assembly, Resolution 48.13, *Communicable disease prevention and control: new, emerging and re-emerging infectious diseases,* was passed (World Health Assembly 1995b). The EID concept appeared at several points in Resolution 48.13, most obviously in its subtitle (see discussion in Chapter 2). Thus World Health Assembly Resolutions 48.7 and 48.13 may be read as beginning the process of harmonizing international health law and WHO organizational practice with the EID concept.

The revision of the IHR (1969) took 10 long years, over the course of which a second, extended critique of the Regulations was produced. In their writings on the IHR (1969), public health experts, social scientists, and legal scholars recapitulated the terms of the early critique, emphasizing how the IHR (1969) were antiquated and outdated. This time, however, their remarks were made as part of analyses about the emerging scope and form of the Regulations' revisions. Many of their arguments took a familiar form. For example, Fidler (1996) and Nicoll et al. (2005) emphasized the increased pace of international trade and travel and the capacity of pathogens to cross national borders undetected as problems that underscored the need to revise the IHR (1969). Noncompliance with maximum health measures and the economic losses in travel and trade that countries faced when they did report were also emphasized by the later critics. For example, Cash and Narasimhan (2000) offered a forceful discussion of the costs to Peru and India of international trade embargoes and tourism restrictions made in response to outbreaks of cholera and plague in their respective territories during the mid-1990s. Echoing Pierre Dorolle's earlier concerns, both Aginam (2002) and Fidler (2004a) emphasized WHO country members' poor compliance with notification requirements as central to the inadequacy of the IHR (1969).

At the same time, much had changed in public health and life sciences' understandings of infectious disease in the 20 years that followed the first period of critique of the IHR (1969). The rapid and widespread circulation of public health concerns about EID, particularly in the global North, provided new grounds for finding fault with the IHR (1969). Controlling EID, which concerned potentiality and emergence in communicable diseases, could not be addressed by the older framework of notification focused on "pestilential diseases" that had dominated international public health law in the 20th century. EID focused a new set of concerns about the IHR (1969) that were expressed with an urgency and with a powerful indictment of the disease list not found in the earlier period of critique.

Multiple critics based outside WHO seized upon the EID concept as a way to find fault with the IHR (1969). Some, such as Lawrence Gostin, the noted scholar of global public health law, argued that the IHR (1969) were limited to diseases initially discussed at the first International Sanitary Conference (1851), which created a narrowness of scope that rendered them "irrelevant for confronting most international threats, ranging from the HIV/AIDS pandemic to SARS" (Gostin 2004b: 2625). Others, such as Plotkin and Kimball (1997: 3), questioned the relevance of the IHR (1969) by contrasting its focus on three infectious diseases to "the long list of known emerging and other infectious diseases that threaten world communities and the threats posed by as yet unknown or unrecognized diseases or syndromes." The concept of EID was thus used to extend the earlier literature's focus on the limited scope of the notification requirements detailed in the IHR (1969). If restricting notification requirements to the disease list was a dated practice in the 1960s and 1970s, then it was doubly so in an age of emerging infections.

The EID concept was further deployed in ways that linked a critique of the IHR as dated with a vision of international infectious disease control as an active and changing terrain. Successfully calling into question the parsimonious logic underlying the reporting requirements of the IHR (1969), the EID concept shattered the presumption of a stable world of infection that could be effectively surveilled by preestablished disease categories. EID displaced the "pestilential diseases of the past" and substituted a shifting and uncertain object that changed understandings of global health surveillance, which could no longer be imagined through the stability of the disease list.

Analytically, EID formed a problematization of the infectious disease list in international health law, posing questions, difficulties, and responses that rendered the IHR (1969) inadequate from the perspective of contemporary thought (Castel 1994; Foucault 1988). The problematization of the infectious disease list by the EID concept was political as well as scientific. It was political in that pressure from the global North was placed on WHO to change its approach to international communicable disease control. The problematization was also scientific, phrased in terms of that which, in principle, could not be listed: potential diseases that did not exist or diseases such as avian influenza that appeared to be close to emerging in humans. The EID concept indexed contemporary genetic microbiology and its conception of the microbial world in constant change, forming new species of microbes and variants of microbes to which humans are susceptible. This conception of the microbial world made obsolete a fixed infectious disease list based on the older assumption of microbial stability.

Two main drafts of the revised IHR were produced during the process of its revision. A first provisional draft was released at the end of January 1998 (WHO 1998). This document was distributed widely to all WHO Member States, interested intergovernmental and nongovernmental organizations, and members of the Committee on International Surveillance of Communicable Diseases (WHO 1998). Even at this early stage of the process, the place of the disease list in international health law was challenged. Among the key proposed changes of the 1998 draft was an expansion of the base of required notification to include all disease outbreaks of international importance. Syndromic surveillance was proposed as the appropriate technique for outbreak detection.

Syndromic surveillance relies on health-related data collected prior to clinical diagnosis; these data are used to indicate the probability of an outbreak that deserves further public health action (CDC 2008). It has been particularly championed as a tool for detecting bioterrorist events because of the speed with which data can be collected. Rather than waiting for clinical diagnoses to occur, syndromic surveillance tracks events such as emergency room admissions, pharmaceutical sales, or changes in the stock market under the assumption that these may indicate an underlying public health emergency (Stoto, Schonlau, & Mariano 2004).

Under a notification system designed for syndromic surveillance, rather than reporting cases of specific infectious diseases, a series of syndromes not requiring specific diagnostic criteria would be subject to report. As expressed by a WHO official we interviewed, following a report of a jaundice syndrome or an acute diarrheal syndrome, decisions would be made regarding the need for further action in relation to the report "rather than automatic publication [in the *Weekly Epidemiological Record*] because the label was cholera" (WHO Interview). A WHO field test of syndromic surveillance in 22 countries prior to 2002 showed that it "was not appropriate for use in the context of a regulatory framework"[11] where the criteria were

> ensuring that only public health risks (usually caused by an infectious agent) that are of urgent international importance are reported under the Regulations; avoiding stigmatization and unnecessary negative impact on international travel and trade of invalid reporting from sources other than Member States, which can have serious economic consequences for countries; making sure that the system is sensitive enough to detect new or re-emerging public health risks.[12]

After WHO had field tested syndromic surveillance and had decided against it, in 2001 it commissioned the Department of Epidemiology of the Swedish Institute for Infectious Disease Control "to establish criteria to define an urgent public health event" (Plotkin, Hardiman, González-Martin, & Rodier 2007: 21) that by 2002 had led to the concept of "public health emergencies of international concern," criteria for their identification, and a draft of a "notification instrument"[13] that with further modification became the basis for the notification algorithm in Annex 2 of the IHR (2005) (Plotkin et al. 2007: 21).

According to Fidler (2004a), after 1998 the revision of the IHR was overshadowed by other international law and public health concerns such as the effect of the World Trade Organization Agreement on Trade-Related Aspects of Intellectual Property Rights on access to essential medicines in the global South. With the SARS outbreak in 2002/2003, however, work on revising the IHR was revitalized. In the wake of SARS, a May 28, 2003 resolution of the World Health Assembly authorized the establishment of an Intergovernmental Working Group open to all Member States to review and recommend a final draft of the IHR for presentation at the World Health Assembly's 2005 annual meeting (World Health Assembly 2003b). The unsettling of the infectious disease list by the EID concept continued in the World Health Assembly Resolution 56.29, *Severe Acute Respiratory Syndrome (SARS)*, which classified SARS as one of the "emerging and re-emerging infectious diseases" that needed international cooperation, better preparedness and response, and improved research (World Health Assembly 2003a). The 56th World Health Assembly also motivated the revision of the IHR in relation to "new risks and threats" formed "from the potential deliberate use of agents for terrorism purposes" (World Health Assembly 2003b).

In January 2004, WHO released a second draft of the revised IHR that was used as the basis for regional WHO consultations conducted that year. The draft was also the subject of comment by Gostin, Fidler, and others who had participated in the second problematization of the IHR (1969) that occurred at the turn of the 21st century. While the provision for syndromic surveillance was dropped, the January 2004 draft advanced the concept of public health risk, a move that displaced the Regulations' focus on the disease list by opening up notification requirements to a wide range of possible threats to public health. The World Health Assembly adopted the Revised International Health Regulations on May 23, 2005 and they entered into force on June 15, 2007.

EID and the Critique of the International Health Law

Our research indicates that internal WHO criticism of the IHR (1969) was not restricted to the early period of critique from 1968 to 1974 but was also a prominent feature of the problematization of the IHR (1969) at the turn of the 21st century. WHO personnel were determined that the revision process of the IHR (1969) would produce a radical break in its notification requirements.

Those we interviewed spoke forcefully about the limitations of the disease list found in the IHR (1969). One participant drew on the notion of stigma to extend a now-familiar basis of concern about obligations to report only named diseases under the IHR (1969):

> Well, it was clear to us that the International Health Regulations were ineffective. They covered only three diseases: cholera, plague, yellow fever. Countries would not report because they got immediately involved in economic sanctions and so nobody reported diseases. Countries didn't report diseases. They didn't want to report cholera because of the stigma. They didn't want to report plague. (WHO Interview)

Another research participant spoke about how a lack of response by WHO to routine reports about "diseases under the Regulations" limited the usefulness of the IHR (1969). Particularly in countries where one or more of the diseases listed in the IHR (1969) was endemic, notification did not generate meaningful responses from WHO. This participant's remarks underscore how, in the field, automatic notification by disease category became decoupled from the international requirement to respond:

> One of the problems we are having with notification of specific diseases is that it's unrelated . . . to the need for WHO to take action either in support of the country or in terms of preventing that spread to other countries. So the fact that in a cholera-endemic country you are notified of

another case of cholera is meaningless in international terms. We know that cholera is there. Nobody should be taking any additional action because of that notification. So countries were not notifying because basically there was no action following notification. There was no result from it, therefore there was no motivation to do it. (WHO Interview)

The disease list of the IHR (1969) thus made little sense to our research participants.

In the late 1990s, WHO staff began to respond to the limitations of the disease list by experimenting with new ways of detecting and responding to outbreaks beyond those mandated by the IHR (1969). The later legal transformations were in effect field tested, as one research participant argued in a passage we quote in extenso here (having already used part of the citation in Chapter 2 in the context of a discussion about the 'world on alert'):

The first thing we did was look at past experiences with Ebola, the plague . . . and we realized that Ebola wasn't under the International Health Regulations and therefore wasn't covered by any framework. And number two, we were doing a pretty poor job in getting information out and getting the response coordinated. So we developed early on a vision for the International Health Regulations which was, we decided we would operationalize the Regulations first rather than revising them from the top down. We needed experience . . . We were always working with a vision which we developed in 1996, which was a world on alert and able to respond to communicable diseases within 24 hours using the most up-to-date communications technology, something to that effect. And that vision always stayed at the forefront as we went through the syndromic and finally fell on a new way. We found syndromic was much too sensitive to get what we needed. And so we went on to the outbreak verification through the Global Alert and Response Network. So we just did it as sort of a vision in front and working towards attaining that vision. (WHO Interview)

As early as 1998, WHO staff in combination with GOARN, a network that they were establishing in the period between 1998 and 2000, had, as we noted in Chapter 3, begun to systematically detect and verify information about outbreaks of infectious diseases—both those that were on the IHR (1969) disease list (Fidler 2003: 286–287) and those, like Ebola hemorrhagic fever, that were not.

The following remarks by another WHO interview participant make clear how the process of revising the IHR (1969) was not only an exercise "on paper" performed by lawyers:

We can't be silly enough or stupid enough to make the assumption that the IHR all of a sudden create the will and the infrastructure to have national systems reporting to us on a 24 hour basis . . . It is my personal belief that the IHR would never have been agreed and WHO would never have been given the mandate, the renewed mandated and expanded mandate we have within the IHR, unless _____ [name] and his colleagues had revolutionized epidemic intelligence with GPHIN, had shown that it is possible to get countries to verify events, had demonstrated that it is possible to build international solidarity for response to such mechanisms like GOARN because what would happen was that the countries were faced with reality. The reality of SARS, flu, of collective responsibility. And what WHO had shown with its partners is that a UN organization could be trusted to build effective surveillance and response means, that we did have the capacities technically and politically to take this issue on. (WHO Interview)

The revision of the IHR (1969) was informed by prior innovations in WHO communicable diseases control activities.

The IHR (2005) in part provided the legal framework for a series of shifts in communicable disease control that had already de facto occurred. At the turn of the 21st century, WHO personnel in the Division of Communicable Diseases, particularly the Department of Communicable Disease Surveillance and Response, were in the process of inventing a new sociotechnical apparatus that would be capable of realizing a world on alert with respect to goals of timeliness in notification and response. They drew on a vision of a world on alert in which real-time information about outbreaks and other events was available to them and in which outbreaks were contained at the source through rapid response coordinated by WHO.

We have shown that the EID concept and security concerns around the intentional spread of pathogens problematized the infectious disease list in the notification requirements of the IHR (1969). During the 1990s the disease list was constructed as an impediment to the formation of a world on alert, which we have previously argued to be a metaphor for global emergency vigilance. The problematization of the infectious disease list through the EID critique showed that the list was an inappropriate way of conceptualizing mandatory notification requirements for global emergency vigilance. The challenge of revising the IHR (1969) was to find legal concepts capable of recognizing a new target of infectious disease control that was characterized by protean potential.

The International Heath Regulations (2005)

The experimental practices of the emergency vigilance apparatus that existed between 1998 and 2003 were recognized in international health law during 2004 and 2005. The IHR (2005) fundamentally redefine the mandatory object of report in international health law through the novel legal concepts of the "public health event" and the "international public health emergency."

These two concepts displace the infectious disease list from international health law. Combined, they produced the legal concept of "events which may constitute a public health emergency of international concern," which defines what is subject to mandatory report under the IHR (2005).

To assist local and national public health officials in interpreting the meaning of public health events, the revised Regulations supply a decision aid in the form of an algorithm, which we refer to as the 'notification algorithm' (see Notification Algorithm, Fig. 4.1, p. 133) and an accompanying guide meant to help public health personnel to interpret what such events might be (see Guide to Completing the Notification Algorithm, Fig. 4.2, p. 134–36). The notification algorithm operationalizes "events which may constitute a public health emergency of international concern" by supplying criteria for evaluating whether or not a given event should be reported to WHO. In the algorithm events are operationalized in terms of three categories: known diseases, emerging diseases, and potential public health events. Together, the algorithm and guide model a form of contextual public health risk assessment, providing a grid of intelligibility for the interpretation of local public health phenomena that require report to WHO.

The shift from a focus on notification of known infectious diseases named in disease lists to notification of events that may constitute public health emergencies of international concern, operationalized through an algorithm and a guide, is significant for international public health in a number of ways. It holds consequences for how global public health security is imagined, for the forms of knowledge that coordinate it, for what is subject to alert, and for how alerts can be entered into knowledge and acted upon. Global emergency vigilance focuses on rapid detection of a range of public health events with a view to containing their international spread. To do so it creates new notification and response obligations for WHO country members while extending the public health role and powers of WHO.

The IHR (2005) reconceptualize mandatory report through a set of relationships established among three related concepts: public health event, public health risk, and public health emergency of international concern. Through these three legal concepts, the IHR (2005) offer up a host of new concerns and potential foci for global health action, redirecting it from the stability of the infectious disease list to a future of multiple and uncertain public health events. In doing so, the IHR (2005) define a more expansive and flexible system of public health action that orients not to the certainty of established disease categories, but to the uncertainty of public health events. In the revised Regulations the disease list is absorbed into new notification requirements that are formulated in relation to public health events and instrumentalized by the notification algorithm and guide. The new Regulations thus mark a fundamental shift from surveillance of the certain to vigilance of public health risk.

The legal concepts of public health event and public health risk are defined in relation to one another in the revised Regulations. They are also defined in terms of a gradation of specificity that moves from the most general concept (event) to the most specific (a public health emergency of international concern). The IHR (2005) define "event" as "a manifestation of disease or an occurrence that creates the potential for disease" (IHR 2005: Art. 1). The relevant manifestations and occurrences encompass a broad range of phenomena including, for example, natural disasters, accidental chemical spills, and the intentional spread of pathogens. The concept of "public health risk" is defined as "the likelihood of an event that may affect adversely the health of human populations, with an emphasis on one which may spread internationally or may present a serious and direct danger" (IHR 2005: Art. 1). Finally, the concept of "public health emergency of international concern" represents the most specific of the three terms. Of all public health events, it is an international public health emergency that is of greatest concern to public health practice in the new IHR. Under the IHR (2005), States Parties are required to report those events which *may* constitute a public health emergency of international concern. A public health emergency of international concern is defined as an extraordinary event determined "to constitute a public health risk to other States through the international spread of disease" and "to potentially require a coordinated international response" (IHR 2005: Art. 1).

The novel concept of a public health emergency of international concern has a number of interesting properties and effects. Most obviously it decouples notification from lists of known diseases. In fact, the concept has such a wide referent that it displaces infectious disease itself as a notification object. Public health emergencies of international concern can include noncommunicable diseases, including those spread internationally by "chemical or radiological agents in products moving in international commerce" (Fidler & Gostin 2006: 86). The target of vigilance is no longer exclusively infectious disease, nor is the practice of vigilance restricted to communicable disease surveillance and control. This marks a fundamental reformulation of public health reasoning.

The concept of a public health emergency of international concern also makes the potential need for WHO response a defining feature of a reportable event. This departs from the notification mechanics of the disease list wherein reporting local outbreaks of cholera, yellow fever, or plague was automatic, regardless of the fact that WHO action rarely occurred in cases of endemic disease. By contrast, a defining principle of what must be reported under the revised IHR—an event that may constitute a public health emergency of international concern—is the need for external assistance to respond and control the event. As such, the IHR (2005) build considerations regarding the possible need for international response into the very notion of what is reportable.

Finally, the concept of a public health emergency of international concern introduces new complexities into the notification requirements of the revised Regulations. Internal to the new legal concepts that specify notification in the IHR (2005) is a distinction between all events and those that might be considered emergencies of international concern. The modulation of event by risk raises the possibility of some events being significant at the level of international transmission and others being not significant. The interpretive dimension built into the central concepts of the revised Regulations, particularly the distinction between all events and emergencies, introduces into notification, forms of judgment and assessment not required under the convention of simple disease-based reporting based on lists.

Under the IHR (2005), WHO holds the sole authority to designate events as public health emergencies of international concern. The declaration of an international health emergency is a speech act that only WHO is authorized to make. In the previous surveillance regime, what we term 'surveillance of the certain,' WHO country members had the authority to report outbreaks of cholera, plague, yellow fever, and before its eradication, smallpox. Under Article 7 of the IHR (1969), WHO sovereign members also determined when an outbreak had ended and were required to report to WHO when an area had become "free from infection." Under the new Regulations, sovereign states only have the obligation to report events that *may* constitute public health emergencies of international concern. The final determination of both whether an event constitutes a public health emergency of international concern and when that event has terminated rests with WHO or, more specifically, with its Director-General.

Our interviews suggest a number of reasons why the concept of event was viewed favorably by WHO officials in their efforts to revise the IHR (1969). They generally viewed the concept as a way to enact the vision of a world on alert guiding the revision process. The concept of event, alongside the notions of public health risk and international public health emergency, had the advantage of bypassing the stasis of the disease list and the non-specificity of syndromic surveillance while encouraging rapid notification. Interview participants partly explained the appeal of event in terms of the everyday currency of the concept. As one official put it, "we actually used that term quite frequently in our daily work" (WHO Interview). The event concept also aligned well with a vision of rapidly identifying outbreaks and other events with a view to their containment. The term was praised for its embrace of "newly recognized" and "relatively sudden occurrences" (WHO Interview). Finally, the broad reach and inclusivity of the concept of event was also positively valued.

One interview participant noted that the term 'event' was partly favored because of its capacity to address security concerns related to the intentional or accidental spread of pathogens. Referring to a meeting held between WHO and representatives of the Ad Hoc Group of States Parties to the Biological Weapons Convention, he noted:

They [members of the Ad Hoc Group] were very interested in making sure the Regulations would also cover diseases that they were concerned about. So we agreed that, yes, these diseases would certainly be important because they were all known diseases. And so that's why we went more to an event, a public health event of importance, using a decision tree mechanism to figure out international public health events so it would cover all these diseases. But we also made it very clear that WHO could not compromise its neutrality by providing specific information to the Biological Weapons Commission, who would provide it to others, nor could we respond at their request. (WHO Interview).

The inherent reach of 'event,' its capacity to capture "a number of things" including emerging infectious diseases and sudden risk factors, was of value to the WHO officials engaged in the IHR revision process. As one interview participant put it, "we chose the term event because it doesn't then say that it's an infectious disease or it's one thing. It allows us to have that broad entry point" (WHO Interview).

While the expansiveness of event as a concept was viewed as an asset by our research participants, it also presented problems. It was one thing to require notification of cholera, plague, and yellow fever, all diseases of known causation, but quite another to require the notification of events that may constitute a public health emergency of international concern. How were such events to be identified globally by public health personnel, and how were they to be conceptualized legally? The concept of public health event represented a dramatic turn from the discursive stability of mandatory reporting in terms of cases of infectious diseases. Incorporating the notion of an event that may be an international public health emergency into the IHR (2005) introduced a significant shift in public health reasoning, one that would need to be fostered and encouraged rather than taken for granted:

I mean this is big. Looking from the public health worker's perspective, this is probably one of the biggest changes in the new IHR. And it's not going to happen overnight. This is going to be a process of learning. And of course that's difficult with an international, legally binding regulation because it sort of enters into force on one day and is in force. And it's actually quite difficult to adapt it to any changing circumstances or learning. So we tried to build that in. (WHO Interview)

The IHR (2005) integrated opportunities for learning and response by WHO country members in view of the much wider and more complex surveillance activities they were obliged to undertake. For example, the Regulations phase-in the new requirements, allowing States Parties 5 years from the time of ratification of the Regulations to fulfill their new notification obligations. A further 2-year extension is possible "in exceptional circumstances" (IHR 2005: Art. 5).[14]

More controversially, the notification of events that may constitute a public health emergency of international concern is associated with the obligation to develop national core capacities in surveillance and response. The IHR (2005) mandates that all WHO country members have national systems with "core capacity requirements for surveillance and response" (IHR 2005: Annex 1, Part A) in place by June 15, 2012 unless individual countries declare otherwise. The IHR (1969) required only that States Parties develop public health capabilities at international ports and airports. The new Regulations make a much stronger intervention into the public health infrastructures of WHO Member States, obliging them to develop a host of domestic surveillance and response capacities. Those requirements are organized in terms of a standard public health institutional hierarchy beginning with local community level and primary public health response levels, proceeding to intermediate public health response levels, and closing with requirements for national levels of response. They include, for example, the capacity to detect unexpected public health events, to report events to the appropriate levels of national health care authority, and to notify WHO of events that may constitute a public health emergency of international concern. In keeping with the temporal demands of a global vigilance regime for a world on alert, they also include the capacity to engage in measures necessary to prevent the domestic and/or international spread of events and the maintenance of an emergency response plan, including the creation of local health care teams to respond to potential public health emergencies of international concern.

The question of where resources to develop core capacities are to come from, especially for counties in the global South, and the potential diversion of resources from other public health priorities to meet the new obligations have made the core capacities an especially controversial new requirement of the IHR (2005; Calain 2007a). Support for the development of national core capacity (surveillance, reporting, notification, verification, response, and collaboration) is mandated under the IHR (2005) to come from WHO and WHO member states (IHR 2005: Annex 1, Art. 3), a provision that transfers the costs of initially developing national core capacity from South to North. The funding of operational costs for ongoing core capacity operations is implicated in North–South issues of resource allocation and governance in the implementation of the IHR (2005) (*PLoS Medicine* Editors 2007).

Beyond phasing-in the IHR's new reporting obligations over time and requiring new surveillance capacities to meet them, the Regulations seek to resolve the problem of requiring mandatory report using a new public health concept unfamiliar to WHO country members through the provision of a particular visual display—the notification algorithm and its guide (Figs. 4.1 and 4.2, p. 133–36). The notification algorithm and the infectious disease list are instances of what Foucault (1976: 79–87) in *The Archeology of Knowledge and the Discourse on Language* called "the statement" (*énoncé*). A statement is composed of signs that are grouped together; it provides the signs with a grid of intelligibility. The signs may be of many kinds: musical, mathematical, graphic, or lingual, among others. A bar is a statement used by musicians; an equation is a statement used by mathematicians. In the IHR (2005), the notification algorithm and the guides are normative statements that organize local and national public health judgment about what to report to WHO as a public health event that may constitute a public health emergency of international concern.

The use of algorithms in medicine dates to the late 1950s, entering medical management from previous uses in cybernetics. They have been employed as devices to promote sequential reasoning in the face of medical uncertainty and popularized as responses that might standardize clinical judgment in the face of evidence showing that some physicians damage patient health through poor decisions (Berg 1995). Most recently, decision aids have been widely promoted as a resource to assist patients in making treatment decisions. In the context of public health, an emerging focus is the use of decision aids to assist people in making decisions about participating in medical screening such as mammography exams and PSA tests for prostate cancer (Barratt, Trevena, Davey, & McCaffery 2004).

The notification algorithm is distinctive as a decision aid in that it seeks to coordinate the decision making of public health officials at a global level. It models a form of sequential binary reasoning designed to assist its readers in making decisions about whether local public health events should be notified to WHO under the Regulations. As such, it can be thought of as a resource for coordinating local public health decisions about whether observed events are instances of what must be reported under the IHR (2005), namely, events that may constitute public health emergencies of international concern.

The notification algorithm takes the form of a decision tree (see Fig. 4.1, p. 133). At the top of the algorithm, three boxes divide public health events into three main types. The left box employs the convention of the disease list, naming diseases that require reporting to WHO. The diseases it lists, however, are not the pestilential diseases of past Regulations, but diseases that are described as unusual or unexpected, including diseases that do not yet exist. The right box also lists diseases, but departs from the conventions of previous disease lists by providing a rationale for their inclusion that can be activated for public health purposes internationally. The diseases listed in the right box are those with a good chance of representing an event that may constitute a public health emergency of international concern because in the past "they have demonstrated the ability to cause serious public health impact and to spread rapidly internationally" (IHR 2005: Annex 2). The right box also includes the innovation of a partial, rather than closed, list that takes the form of examples of a higher-order concept, namely diseases "that are of special national or regional concern." The lists of diseases appearing in the right box are distinguishable from previous disease lists in international health law because they are conceptually tied to the organizing concept of "events that may constitute a public health emergency of international concern." The notification mechanics prompted by local instances of the diseases or types of diseases listed in the right box also departs from the convention of past disease lists. Rather than triggering immediate notification, they activate the decision tree. Finally, the middle box is the site in the algorithm where the new concept of event introduced by the IHR (2005) has its most immediate discursive presence. The middle box departs from past notification conventions by absenting disease names and directing attention to a wide range of public health events of potential international concern. In the context of the IHR (2005), 'event' is not an infectious disease-specific concept. The relevant events *can* include outbreaks of infectious diseases, but they can include much else. The middle box of the notification algorithm includes infectious diseases not listed in the left or right boxes, noncommunicable diseases that may cross national boundaries, and public health events with known or unknown causes that may lead to the international transmission of diseases. Local instances of diseases or events that fall under the middle box also trigger use of the decision tree.

The notification algorithm is structured as a decision tree organized in terms of a descending sequence of four questions, each of which can be answered affirmatively or negatively. Progress through the decision tree is organized in terms of a yes/no response to each successive question. The questions in sequence are: (1) Is the public health impact of the event serious? (2) Is the event unusual or unexpected? (3) Is there a significant risk of international spread? (4) Is there a significant risk of international travel or trade restriction? The notification algorithm is accompanied by a guide to assist readers in reaching their yes/no decisions (see Fig. 4.2.1, 4.2.2 and 4.2.3, Guide to Completing the Notification Algorithm). For each of the four questions that appear in the notification algorithm, the guide offers suggested supplementary questions that the reader might pose in reaching a decision. For example, to answer the first question (Is the public health impact of the event serious?) the guide invites readers to ask the following questions: "Is the number of cases/and or number of deaths for this type of event large for the given place, time or population?"; "Has the event the potential to have a high public health impact?"; and "Is external assistance needed to detect, investigate, respond and control the current event, or prevent new cases?" For three of the four central questions of the notification algorithm, the guide also provides examples of circumstances and events that represent affirmative responses. Thus "cases reported among health staff" and an "event in an area with high population density" are offered by the guide as examples of events with the potential to have a high impact on public health.

The notification algorithm and guide are textual devices that seek to coordinate and streamline the notification process by assisting WHO country members to determine which public health events should be reported.

DECISION INSTRUMENT FOR THE ASSESSMENT AND NOTIFICATION
OF EVENTS THAT MAY CONSTITUTE A PUBLIC HEALTH EMERGENCY
OF INTERNATIONAL CONCERN

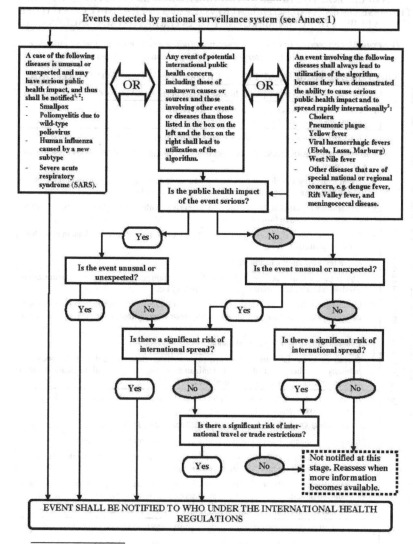

Figure 4.1   Notification algorithm.

Comment: The notification algorithm acts as a decision aid for reporting events rather than cases, the unit of report under the IHR (1969). Whereas previous international health law oriented public health practice to notification of a small number of known diseases, the notification algorithm has a threefold division of events: known infectious diseases, emerging infectious diseases, and potential public health events. This algorithm supplies criteria to assist local/national public health personnel in evaluating whether or not a given event should be reported to WHO.

Source: IHR (2005): 43, Annex 2.

EXAMPLES FOR THE APPLICATION OF THE DECISION INSTRUMENT FOR THE ASSESSMENT AND NOTIFICATION OF EVENTS THAT MAY CONSTITUTE A PUBLIC HEALTH EMERGENCY OF INTERNATIONAL CONCERN

The examples appearing in this Annex are not binding and are for indicative guidance purposes to assist in the interpretation of the decision instrument criteria.

DOES THE EVENT MEET AT LEAST TWO OF THE FOLLOWING CRITERIA?

	I. Is the public health impact of the event serious?
	1. *Is the number of cases and/or number of deaths for this type of event large for the given place, time or population?*
	2. *Has the event the potential to have a high public health impact?*
	THE FOLLOWING ARE EXAMPLES OF CIRCUMSTANCES THAT CONTRIBUTE TO HIGH PUBLIC HEALTH IMPACT:
	✓ Event caused by a pathogen with high potential to cause epidemic (infectiousness of the agent, high case fatality, multiple transmission routes or healthy carrier).
	✓ Indication of treatment failure (new or emerging antibiotic resistance, vaccine failure, antidote resistance or failure).
	✓ Event represents a significant public health risk even if no or very few human cases have yet been identified.
	✓ Cases reported among health staff.
	✓ The population at risk is especially vulnerable (refugees, low level of immunization, children, elderly, low immunity, undernourished, etc.).
	✓ Concomitant factors that may hinder or delay the public health response (natural catastrophes, armed conflicts, unfavourable weather conditions, multiple foci in the State Party).
	✓ Event in an area with high population density.
	✓ Spread of toxic, infectious or otherwise hazardous materials that may be occurring naturally or otherwise that has contaminated or has the potential to contaminate a population and/or a large geographical area.
	3. *Is external assistance needed to detect, investigate, respond and control the current event, or prevent new cases?*
	THE FOLLOWING ARE EXAMPLES OF WHEN ASSISTANCE MAY BE REQUIRED:
	✓ Inadequate human, financial, material or technical resources – in particular:
	– insufficient laboratory or epidemiological capacity to investigate the event (equipment, personnel, financial resources);
	– insufficient antidotes, drugs and/or vaccine and/or protective equipment, decontamination equipment, or supportive equipment to cover estimated needs;
	– existing surveillance system is inadequate to detect new cases in a timely manner.
	IS THE PUBLIC HEALTH IMPACT OF THE EVENT SERIOUS? **Answer "yes" if you have answered "yes" to questions 1, 2 or 3 above.**

(Left vertical heading: Is the public health impact of the event serious?)

Figure 4.2.1 Guide to completing the notification algorithm.

Comment: The Guide to Completing the Notification Algorithm conceptually coordinates local decision making by public health officials with the notification requirements of the IHR (2005). They do this by supplying and ordering questions to assess local events in terms of their likelihood of being events that may constitute a public health emergency of international concern. The guide and the notification algorithm format public health judgment as a practice of qualitative, contextually sensitive risk assessment.

Source: IHR (2005): 45–46, Annex 2.

	II. Is the event unusual or unexpected?
Is the event unusual or unexpected?	4. *Is the event unusual?* THE FOLLOWING ARE EXAMPLES OF UNUSUAL EVENTS: ✓ The event is caused by an unknown agent or the source, vehicle, route of transmission is unusual or unknown. ✓ Evolution of cases more severe than expected (including morbidity or case-fatality) or with unusual symptoms. ✓ Occurrence of the event itself unusual for the area, season or population. 5. *Is the event unexpected from a public health perspective?* THE FOLLOWING ARE EXAMPLES OF UNEXPECTED EVENTS: ✓ Event caused by a disease/agent that had already been eliminated or eradicated from the State Party or not previously reported.
	IS THE EVENT UNUSUAL OR UNEXPECTED? **Answer "yes" if you have answered "yes" to questions 4 or 5 above.**

	III. Is there a significant risk of international spread?
Is there a significant risk of international spread?	6. *Is there evidence of an epidemiological link to similar events in other States?* 7. *Is there any factor that should alert us to the potential for cross border movement of the agent, vehicle or host?* THE FOLLOWING ARE EXAMPLES OF CIRCUMSTANCES THAT MAY PREDISPOSE TO INTERNATIONAL SPREAD: ✓ Where there is evidence of local spread, an index case (or other linked cases) with a history within the previous month of: – international travel (or time equivalent to the incubation period if the pathogen is known); – participation in an international gathering (pilgrimage, sports event, conference, etc.); – close contact with an international traveller or a highly mobile population. ✓ Event caused by an environmental contamination that has the potential to spread across international borders. ✓ Event in an area of intense international traffic with limited capacity for sanitary control or environmental detection or decontamination.
	IS THERE A SIGNIFICANT RISK OF INTERNATIONAL SPREAD? **Answer "yes" if you have answered "yes" to questions 6 or 7 above.**

Figure 4.2.2 Guide to completing the notification algorithm.

When moving through the notification algorithm and/or its complementary guide, affirmative answers to two of the four central questions translate local events into the discursive terms of the IHR (2005) as notifiable events, namely those "which may constitute a public health emergency of international concern." A lack of any affirmative response or only one affirmative response generates an end result of no notification but leaves open the possibility of later notification through repetition of the decision exercise when additional information becomes available.

	IV. Is there a significant risk of international travel or trade restrictions?
Risk of international restrictions?	8. *Have similar events in the past resulted in international restriction on trade and/or travel?*
	9. *Is the source suspected or known to be a food product, water or any other goods that might be contaminated that has been exported/imported to/from other States?*
	10. *Has the event occurred in association with an international gathering or in an area of intense international tourism?*
	11. *Has the event caused requests for more information by foreign officials or international media?*
	IS THERE A SIGNIFICANT RISK OF INTERNATIONAL TRADE OR TRAVEL RESTRICTIONS? Answer "yes" if you have answered "yes" to questions 8, 9, 10 or 11 above.

States Parties that answer "yes" to the question whether the event meets any two of the four criteria (I-IV) above, shall notify WHO under Article 6 of the International Health Regulations.

Figure 4.2.3   Guide to completing the notification algorithm.

The notification algorithm and guide are interpretive devices that conceptually coordinate the local decision making of public health officials into terms that can generate events that are meaningful in terms of the notification requirements stipulated in the IHR (2005). They do this by supplying and ordering a host of questions that assess local events in terms of their likelihood of being events that may constitute a public health emergency of international concern. This involves asking questions about whether events pose a significant risk to public health at an international level. Thus, readers are enjoined to consider whether the event is occurring in settings associated with high volumes of international traffic or where surveillance and response resources are weak, whether the route of transmission is unusual or unknown, the extent to which treatment failure is indicated or the affected risk population is especially vulnerable, and so on. The notification algorithm and its accompanying guide thus serve to format public health judgment as a practice of qualitative, contextually sensitive risk assessment.

The IHR (2005) offer an example of the incorporation of risk as a legal concept within international public health law. The effect of this incorporation is to undergird a conceptual break in the organization of global public health notification from a closed, disease-based form to one that constructs public health events as both known and unknown. But mandatory reporting under the IHR (2005) also draws on earlier forms of public health reasoning, particularly those that would assess phenomena contextually. The sought-after form of public health judgment is elaborated in the following interview participant's comments about the guide and notification algorithm:

> The instrument is asking them to assess not just the diagnosis—if you have that, that's very useful—but also the context in which the event

is occurring. Is this something that is going to spread because it's in a major city? Is it affecting a transportation hub? Is it happening on a border so we should be talking with the neighbors? Is it happening during the World Cup, you know, where there are people from all over the world here? You know, taking the context into account. Is this so unusual from what we had last year? Are people dying from this disease when last year it was mild?. . . . So we tried to build in those thought processes into those four questions and the indicators that are listed underneath that. And they are not intended to be exhaustive or completely rigid. The Regulations also say that if you can't come out with a clear answer when you use this, consult with WHO. So it allows flexibility, but it also provides guidance as to the kind of issues that should be considered when deciding that this is of international significance or this is very unusual or very serious. (WHO Interview)

WHO officials were well aware of the shifts in the mechanics of notification represented by the revised IHR when they devised the notification algorithm and guide to support local decision making. The forms of risk assessment and overall judgment promoted through the notification algorithm and the guide of the IHR (2005) are contextually based. The practical success of the IHR (2005) and, by extension, of global public health vigilance more broadly, depends on the ability of local public health personnel to successfully report events that may be public health emergencies of international concern.

Decision making under the notification requirements of the IHR (1969) was relatively simple. Considered abstractly, notification was accomplished through recognizing local instances of one or more elements of a set of disease categories. Notification involved recognizing a local outbreak as a manifestation of one of the four infectious diseases upon which, ideally, automatic reporting to WHO was to follow. The work of producing the notification of cholera, plague, yellow fever, or smallpox involved medical diagnosis and epidemiological fieldwork, but with a clear relation between type (the disease) and token (the case). The decision-making mechanics of notification under the revised Regulations are a far more complex form of practical reasoning. Events that may constitute public health emergencies of international concern only come into being as a consequence of a decision-making process that engages contextual forms of public health reasoning about a given event's risk to international public health.

The wide empirical referent for events that may be international public health emergencies, which extends well beyond instances of a static disease list, and the very discursive novelty of the term within global public health circles present notification problems that the algorithm and guide seek to address. The incorporation of these two related textual devices in the IHR (2005) offers an important example of how the revised Regulations engage text/action relations of a different order than those created by the IHR (1969). As noted in Chapter 1, the notion that texts are active constituents of social relations, particularly those relations that govern contemporary society, is a feature of Smith's work on the social organization of knowledge. The many critiques of the IHR (1969) as hopelessly behind the times can in part be interpreted as a manifestation of its sluggish text/action relations. The IHR (1969) was largely ignored in the field, and among global public health officials it could not generate observance of the notification requirements or maximum health measures that were its two central requirements.

As discussed earlier in this chapter, the reasons for noncompliance with the IHR (1969) are complex and only partly related to the limitations of the disease list. Whether greater compliance will be forthcoming for the notification requirements of the IHR (2005) remains to be seen. The IHR (2005) provided legal authorization for a vigilance regime characterized by near real-time response to a wide range of globally significant public health events that come into knowledge at WHO with newfound speed. As one interview participant put it, under conditions of global health vigilance and a world on alert, it would be "honorable and the norm for a country to report rather than to not report" (WHO Interview). The challenge that outbreak detection brings to sovereign control over the knowledge of public health events and ameliorative responses to the economic repercussions of notification are among the factors relevant to the realization of these new notification norms of report. While the revised IHR cannot themselves secure such norms, they are distinguished from the IHR (1969) by their seeking to intervene in the text/action relations of notification in new ways. The algorithm and guide provided by the IHR (2005) are important examples of textual devices that seek to project into the field precisely those forms of public health reasoning that secure the forms of notification required of a global health vigilance regime.

Conclusion

After more than a century of organizing notification requirements for international infectious disease control in terms of fixed, listed diseases, the IHR (2005) replaced the infectious disease list with the concept of an event that may constitute a public health emergency of international concern. We have argued that the displacement of infectious disease by international public health emergency and of the case by the event were motivated by the restructuring of international communicable disease control as a vigilance system that constantly monitors the earth for signs of trouble and seeks to intervene before they become catastrophic. The incorporation of the 'event' concept within the IHR (2005), and particularly the creation of the legal concept of an "event which may constitute a public health emergency of international concern," made official reporting requirements consistent with shifts in infectious disease control practice that had begun at WHO in the late 1990s. The concept of 'public health event' also increased the empirical reach of what became subject to notification under international health law, making official reporting requirements compatible not only with EID detection, but also with chemical, radiological, and environmental disasters, and the deliberate and accidental spread of pathogens. Continuing to conceptualize the detection of and response to international public health events as falling within communicable disease control made little sense; and thus, as we will show in the next chapter, communicable disease control came to be encompassed by the novel concept of 'public health security.'

Operationalizing the new practices of mandatory report through the notification algorithm and its accompanying guide helped resolve the problem of establishing an international legal structure of notification based on a novel concept that was unfamiliar to local public health officials. The algorithm and guide projected into a global field of public health action the forms of judgment required to secure local reports of the form of events the IHR (2005) demand. It became possible in principle for previously unknown diseases to be reported to the watchful apparatus of WHO.

Making the IHR (1969) compatible with the need for real-time detection of and response to international public health emergencies necessitated a deep change in the legal conceptualization of communicable disease control in international health law. Global emergency vigilance required that the sovereign states that were WHO members agree to international law that would weaken sovereign power over information pertaining to potential international public health emergencies. The IHR (2005) harmonized international public health law with global emergency vigilance by taking apart the postcolonial settlement in international communicable disease control that had extended the Euro-American legal convention that infectious disease report was a sovereign matter to newly independent states during the late 1940s and 1950s. In the following chapter we will examine how emergency vigilance changed the terrain of international politics in health by transforming WHO from an interstate organization to a global one with powers in public health emergencies that exceed sovereign power.

Most scholarly writing on the International Health Regulations is organized by strong normative commitments. The central trajectory of writing has moved from earlier critiques of the IHR (1969) to more recent commentary that generally praises a number of innovations that have been incorporated into the IHR (2005). Of course, the most recent discussion of the revised Regulations is not without critical commentary. Some authors have called into question the continued legacy of colonialism under the IHR (2005) and have noted that new surveillance arrangements will likely benefit the developed world while placing on developing countries new surveillance burdens that strain already limited resources (J.M. Wilson, von Tigerstrom, & McDougall 2008; Calain 2007a). Others have posed concerns about the growing association of public health with national security and raised questions about how perceived bioterrorist threats render the global health surveillance apparatus vulnerable to the pursuit of national security interests (Calain 2007b). For our part, we have sought to register with greater clarity than has been done thus far the significance of conceptual innovations and changes in knowledge for emerging forms of global public health vigilance.

5 A World on Alert
Emergency Vigilance in Global Biopolitics

This chapter differs from the preceding ones in that it is primarily a work of social and political theory. The previous chapters were more typical of a sociology of health and illness in that they were primarily empirical with social scientific inductive analysis. For the most part, social theory and empirical research overlap little, particularly in the field of health, which has a strongly applied character.

Theory subjects concepts and arguments to close deliberation, fore-grounding its own concepts and arguments for examination; it reflects on the worlds that science and medicine are constituting. As many simply want to get on with the job that theory subjects to reflection, social and political theory will inevitably be perceived as a pest. Yet it might also be observed that social theorists often begin their reflections on the basis of a present known only from the morning newspaper, that owl of Minerva. Overall our work in the present book is fundamentally theoretico-empirical as we needed to do empirical research in order to know what it was we were to theorize. Theoretico-empirical work has three levels: the empirical, the analytic, and the theoretical. We proceed to the theoretical now.

Global emergency vigilance represents an epistemological shift in public health reasoning that led to an historical break in which WHO was con-stituted as a suprasovereign power. Ours is a seeming Hobbesian tale of WHO's sovereign country members fearing lawless and anarchic pathogens so much that they decided to save themselves from the state of nature by enhancing the power of WHO as an interstate organization, transforming WHO into a power over and above themselves to know about and deal with international public health emergencies. Yet in that state of nature, sovereign states were not in a relation of equivalence. It was a curious state of nature that was already characterized by political division, and its tran-scendence was accomplished by the strong diplomacy of the USA and its allies acting as a power bloc.

As an epistemological shift, emergency vigilance has the following char-acteristics. First, the target of international public health action is transposed from infectious disease to international public health emergency. By target we mean the main antagonist that WHO is given in international health law: how the main public health threat is conceived. A target is conceptually constructed (Bourdieu, Chamboredon, & Passeron 1968/1991: 33–35). It indicates what global public health must act on, what its primary mandate is. WHO gathers information about public health events in order to identify those that are international public health emergencies—its current target—as cholera, plague, smallpox, and yellow fever were the targets of international public health action under the IHR (1969). Second, emergency vigilance is concerned with the potential, the emerging, and the actual, whereas the prior period of international communicable disease control dealt only with the actual. Third, emergency vigilance is characterized by the reflexive coordination of causal (case-based) and noncausal (event-based) knowledge of public health events. Fourth, emergency vigilance has the temporal standard of what is called 'real time' or 'near real time.' Real time presupposes the effective establishment of global, synchronized time, as distinct from the discontinuity between local time and international time that existed in WHO's work until the late 1990s. Prior to the formation of real time, the local chronology of outbreak and WHO's narration of it were asynchronous, that is, they occurred in separate temporal orders. Fifth, emergency vigilance is characterized by an expansion of the scope of international communicable disease control to include the public health aspects of international disasters (chemical, environmental, industrial) and weapons (biological, chemical, nuclear and radiological) incidents. Unlike prior international public health, emergency vigilance is securitized.

After characterizing emergency vigilance as an epistemological shift, we move to consider the reconstitution of the political in global biopolitics that took place in the name of containing international public health emergencies. The revision of the IHR (2005) overcame the sovereignty problem in international health law—the location of the ultimate place of power in the sovereign—by giving WHO what amounted to an informal power of sanction associated with the announcement of international public health emergencies. The IHR (2005) also conferred on WHO global powers that could be exercised without sovereign consent under specified conditions. Although many have written about the recent emergence of WHO as a power above the sovereign, and our present account in particular owes much to David Fidler's (2004b: 132–145) analysis of WHO's powers to issue global alerts and to use nongovernmental epidemiological information as post-Westphalian, the specificity of our analysis lies in linking these powers—which amount to an emancipation of epidemiological information about public health events beyond sovereignty—to the epistemological shift associated with global emergency vigilance: its target, its relation to the potential, its articulation of surface and depth knowledge, its real-time temporal standard, and its securitization. The IHR (2005) did not simply give WHO powers; it gave juridical form to a preexisting epistemological shift.

In the concluding section of this chapter, we object to theorizing global biopolitics purely in terms of governance and conceptualize it as having three aspects: a level of governance, one of sovereignty, and a suprasovereign level organized around a symbolic conception of a common fate in global public health. Our general intent here is to fashion a conception of biopolitics wherein the political is irreducible both to the governmental and to the sovereign. Expansive concepts of governance that elide the political cannot think through questions of representation, membership, recognition, inclusion, exclusion, distribution, and the formation of the political scene where division and contestation occur (Fraser 2005). Nor can the spread of governmental forms without political accountability at the global level receive an adequate diagnosis if the political is reduced to governance. There is much at stake in the distinction between the political and the governmental in global biopolitics, as elsewhere.

From the perspective of our case study, global biopolitics appears as an emancipation of public health knowledge[1] from sovereign power, although we do not project this as a general theory of globalization. Global emergency vigilance represents an epistemological shift in public health thinking that required a break from previous forms of international communicable disease control that were under ultimate sovereign control. The emancipation of public health knowledge pertaining to emergencies first took the form of what we have termed 'pure governance' as WHO personnel worked to create institutional practices and knowledge relations that would be capable of realizing the epistemological character of the world on alert, the strategic plan for the WHO Division of Emerging and other Communicable Diseases Surveillance and Control (discussed in Chapter 2). After emergency vigilance as a governance form had been stabilized, it was given juridical form in the reconstitution of WHO as a (limited) suprasovereign power as distinct from its prior form as an interstate organization. Pure governance exists in the space between a law that has been declared obsolete and the passing of a new law that will bring its actions within the sphere of right. Against the tendency in contemporary scholarship (Benoist 2008; Ong 2006) that would interpret contemporary international/global politics as primarily characterized by states of exception, we offer pure governance as an equivocal state not reducible to the state of exception, in the context of a case study (global emergency vigilance) where governance outside the law was later brought within international law.

We are aware that there is an objection in the wings to our considerations of biopolitics. We have heard it often. Some might protest that WHO governance in the area of international public health emergencies responds to purely empirical, scientific problems. WHO in turn might be interpreted as a suprapolitical body with stakes so imperative that they lie above any political process. Emergency vigilance would then appear as purely humanitarian and beyond politics. If so, our writing would be vitiated.

This objection relies on three postulates: science represents reality; public health governance stands for science; the political ought to align with science and public health in relation to microbial imperatives. These claims ultimately rest on the supposition that science is the mirror of nature.

First, the postulate that science represents the real is based on an empiricist theory of knowledge. Empiricism understands words to be surface representations of deep causal processes within things; knowledge represents the immanence of things, and does so without addition. This does not work very well for global emergency vigilance as it is rather hard to characterize potential diseases if they have never previously existed. The growth of governance oriented to the emerging and potential is one in which representation anticipates rather than repeats what exists.

Second, public health governance of any kind does not simply reproduce scientific fact because governance bridges between the normative and factual (Singer & Weir 2006: 457; Weir 2008: 377–378). Governmental knowledge seeks to make normative interventions, to effect the right disposition of persons and things. Public health governance links what ought to be on the basis of knowledge taken to be descriptive of what is or what might potentially exist. Governance is not a simple representation of things; rather, it uses empirical knowledge to change that which exists.

Third, the formulation of global emergency vigilance as a wise humanitarian abdication of the political is ignorant of the history of the political alliances through which that vigilance apparatus was constituted. The push for the formation of global emergency vigilance came from the global North in response to the IOM's problematization of domestic and international communicable disease control through the EID concept. Public health emergencies and endemic diseases require differing kinds of public health response; once a disease such as HIV/AIDS has become prevalent, emergency management measures are ineffective. The political question then necessarily arises as to appropriate resource allocation across differing aspects of public health programming: which expenditures have maximum health benefits, how much should be spent, where the budget should come from. Our point here is that the political does not vanish in the face of public health emergencies. The meaning of microbes is constituted in a politically divided world.

Global Emergency Vigilance as an Epistemological Shift

We here consider global emergency vigilance as an epistemological shift from prior international communicable disease control at WHO that focuses on the target of international public health action, the relation between deep (causal) and surface (associationist) knowledge, the temporal standard to which public health knowledge is held, and its relation to security.

A) The Target of Public Health Action

Emergency vigilance as an epistemological shift was from the first articulated to political pressure for deep changes in domestic and international public health governance. It began as a U.S. political initiative to change the USA's own domestic public health system, an initiative made in the name of controlling new, emerging, and reemerging infectious diseases (see Chapter 2). Between 1993 and 1995 the EID concept was deployed by sovereign states of the global North to demand that WHO refashion its system of communicable disease control. This political initiative was led by a combination of public health personnel and life scientists (epidemiologists, geneticists, virologists, microbiologists, and others) who advocated strengthening international infectious disease control.

Global emergency vigilance has a breadth of target that is historically unprecedented in international communicable disease control. As we saw in Chapter 4, during the period from the ISR (1951) to the problematization of the IHR (1969) in the mid-1990s, the target of mandatory report to WHO was conceptualized as infectious disease, more precisely those infectious diseases listed in international health law. Under the IHR (1969) these were cholera, plague, smallpox (prior to its eradication), and yellow fever. WHO country members were required under international law to report cases of these diseases to WHO, and WHO was also legally obligated to halt their international transmission.

The period from roughly 1996 to 2001 was one of experimentation in international communicable disease control at WHO: the beginning of global emergency vigilance. During the period from 1995 to 2000 the target of vigilance was initially formulated as outbreak. One sees this in the names chosen during the late 1900s for the vigilance apparatus: WHO's Outbreak Alert and Response Operations Team, Outbreak Verification Team, GOARN (Global Outbreak Alert and Response Network). GPHIN and ProMED-mail were called online early warning outbreak detection systems. Although formally synonymous with 'epidemic,' in actual use 'outbreak' was and is treated as an interval at the start of an epidemic when quick and timely public health intervention might still be able to contain it. Outbreak also applied, following its standard 20th century usage in public health epidemiology, to both communicable and noncommunicable diseases (see discussion in Chapter 1), but during the mid 1990s outbreak was extended to include bioweapons incidents. ProMED-mail was developed from the first to detect bioweapons use. By the late 1990s 'outbreak' had in practice been stretched far beyond its formal public health application to diseases.

The outbreak concept continued in use throughout the first decade of the 21st century, but it was partially displaced by the concept of international public health emergency. Unlike the concept of outbreak, which is formally restricted to diseases, 'emergency' includes diseases but extends beyond them. This would initially appear at variance with the scope of the IHR (2005), which is defined in terms of disease: "to prevent, protect against, control and provide a public health response to the international spread of disease" (IHR 2005: Art. 2). Disease is, however, given a special legal sense in the IHR (2005) to include medical conditions: "'disease' means an illness or medical condition, irrespective of origin or source, that presents or could prevent significant harm to humans" (IHR 2005: Art.1). "Medical condition" is not defined in the IHR (2005). Disease in this legal sense is close to 'dis-ease,' or 'unease,' rather than the specialized meaning of disease that has obtained in medicine since the beginning of the 19th century (Bynum 1993a: 348–353).

With the concept of international public health emergency, the IHR (2005) broke with infectious disease as the target of all previous international health law. An international public health emergency consists of an illness or medical condition affecting population(s) that has spread or threatens to spread internationally, either because control measures won't work, the sovereign state involved lacks the relevant control capacity, or the danger of international transmission in a given case requires urgent action (IHR 2005: Art. 11). The international public health emergency concept thus extends far beyond outbreak into mass disasters affecting human health that cross international boundaries: intentional and nonintentional biological, chemical, environmental, industrial, or radiological disasters. The public health effects of such disasters include not only disease in the medical sense, but also health consequences beyond disease. Chemical disasters may poison people without causing disease, and radiological disasters may kill people long prior to the onset of thyroid cancer.

The concept of international public health emergencies produces a target for global emergency vigilance that has substantial similarities with the EID concept. Both project a threefold target, although the public health emergency concept has a broader application to all diseases, not simply infectious ones, and to medical conditions. International public health emergency has a tripartite target that consists of diseases and conditions that are existent, emergent, and potential.[2] The potential is conceived not as the actualization of something that already exists, but as the actualization of that which has not yet entered being. Potentiality has the additional capacity to enter actuality or not to do so. Given the conceptualization of international public health emergencies as including emerging and potential phenomena, public health knowledge is by implication necessarily incomplete. For the purposes of global emergency vigilance, detection must in principle be designed to provide sensitivity to diseases/conditions previously unknown, whether due to geopolitical ignorance of communicable diseases found in the global South or because a disease has only recently been actualized from potential microbial being.

Emergency vigilance requires watchfulness over a target that consists of the actual, the emergent, and the potential. It differs in fundamental ways from the infectious disease lists that were found in international health law from the International Sanitary Convention (1892) to the IHR (1969). The disease list was a statement addressed to the present, the known, and the certain, and thus lacked the capacity to formulate public health action in relation to infectious diseases just coming into existence and those still in the realm of the potential. Emergencies are not confined to infectious diseases, indeed not to any disease. More fundamentally, the tripartite conceptual target of emergency vigilance troubles the relation between words and things that characterized the disease list in previous international health law and practice. The disease list is part of a system of representation characterized by very complicated things/subjects that have interior processes known through and represented by words, formulae, and other signs. The name of a disease is taken to mirror the immanence of deep processes external to and preexisting representation.

In the tripartite target of emergency vigilance things have become much more complicated as the unusual, the unknown, and the unexpected proliferate. Words enter into a distance from things and become a rough set of responsible and reasonable decision principles for standardizing international judgment about the known and the unknown. The disease list in international law had assumed that definitive diagnosis was possible—a relation of certainty between words and the things that were making some people sick with cholera or yellow fever or smallpox. This relation of certainty is, of course, dependent on the presence of health care personnel and laboratories, access to which is stratified by position in the global economic order, but this is a matter of justice and the point under discussion is a small epistemological one: The disease list names known diseases that in principle may be identified in patients. The conceptual target of emergency vigilance establishes three relations between words and things: (1) a relation of certainty wherein words identify diseases/emergencies with known causes; (2) a relation of uncertainty wherein words have a complex relation to things that do not quite exist, but which may emerge from known causes (e.g., SARS and smallpox) or from causes that may reasonably be anticipated (e.g., H5N1, avian influenza); and (3) a relation of potentiality that at its limit has no words for diseases/conditions wherein causes do not exist and have not been imagined.

B) The Coordination of Surface and Depth Knowledge

Emergency vigilance is characterized by the coexistence of depth and surface knowledge acting jointly. Depth knowledge begins by dividing a phenomenon of interest into exterior and interior, and it explains the exterior in terms of the interior. Clinical medicine, first formed in the early 19th century, is an example of depth knowledge; it links signs and symptoms visible on the body's surface with events found in the body's interior. Surface knowledge is not organized in terms of a division between interior and exterior; it does not operate in terms of deep inner causes, seeking rather to identify surface patterns or relays in complex networks (Deleuze 1995).

During the second half of the 20th century a variety of surface knowledges entered medicine, notably risk in clinical practice (Armstrong 1995; Weir 2006: 57–65) and, it has been argued, molecular medicine (Rose 2007). Although one particular form of surface knowledge, online early warning outbreak detection, has been the focus of our analysis in this book, a number of other event-based monitoring systems were either in use or were being devised at the turn of the 21st century. These included syndromic surveillance systems that attempt to recognize outbreaks by identifying clusters of data, typically consumer purchases and health care system use. Our present is characterized by the growth of biosurveillance methods seeking early warning of outbreak and other events: surface knowledge. In the first decade of the 21st century a general field of early warning outbreak detection called biosurveillance has been constituted (Wagner et al. 2001; Wagner 2006: 3). Certain biosurveillance techniques track disease in wildlife and domestic animals with the goal to detect outbreaks prior to their appearance as cases in humans. Other surveillance techniques relevant to public health analyze climate reports and geospatial data. Public health scholarship contrasts biosurveillance techniques based on event monitoring with what is called 'traditional' infectious disease surveillance based on case reports of disease (Green & Kaufman 2002: 503; Sosin 2003: 247): a contrast between surface and depth within surveillance itself.

Early warning outbreak detection, the systematic analysis of informal sources, is a surface knowledge. It differs from earlier forms of epidemiological surveillance in being event based rather than case based.[3] This form of outbreak detection is sourced in nonmedical, unofficial, digitized information rather than on diagnostic reports about pathologies occurring in the depths of the body, and it uses the digitized information of events as the basis for issuing alerts. Case-based surveillance is dependent on diagnostic information; it is a depth knowledge based on linking signs and symptoms to interior pathologies. The massive growth of surface, event-based monitoring has, however, also been associated with demands for better case-based surveillance. Surface does not displace depth in global emergency vigilance; they coexist and interact.

In comparison with early warning outbreak detection, the depth knowledge of case-based surveillance is clearly the older method of detection, dating to the mid-1950s. In the first half of the 20th century, the term 'surveillance' in public health meant the observation of individuals who had come into contact with those having infectious disease. The movements of the contacts were not restricted unless they showed symptoms, and then they were placed in isolation (Langmuir 1963, 1976; Thacker 2000: 11; Thacker & Berkelman 1988: 166). Alexander Langmuir, the chief epidemiologist at what was then called the Communicable Disease Center (now the Centers for Disease Control and Prevention [CDC]) during the 1950s and 1960s, is credited with changing the meaning of surveillance by applying it to populations rather than individuals. Langmuir extended surveillance to noninfectious diseases and tied surveillance data to action through information dissemination and alliances with government (Thacker & Gregg 1996: S26). Early warning outbreak detection systems broke with Langmuir's form of national surveillance and its forms of data collection that were primarily based on the case report and substituted the event in its place. GPHIN and ProMED-mail were devised to have a global reach by their use of online, unofficial data sources that for the most part escaped national control.

Emergency vigilance as an epistemological shift is marked by the systemic incorporation of surface knowledge within global public health reasoning. However, surface knowledge does not result in the displacement of depth knowledge in domestic and global public health. Rather, surface and depth knowledge coexist and interact, increasing the numbers of outbreaks and emergencies detected. By way of example, one can point to the fact that under the IHR (2005) the national core capacity requirements for surveillance and response specify that the first level of surveillance (local community or primary health care) is to be able to report all "essential information," which is interpreted to include "clinical descriptions, laboratory results, sources and type of risk, numbers of human cases and deaths, conditions affecting the spread of disease and the health measures employed" (IHR 2005: Annex 1, Art. 4). Event-based monitoring does not displace case-based surveillance in global vigilance. Surface and depth act in tandem.

C) Temporal Standard

Global emergency vigilance has a distinctive temporal organization that is oriented to the normative standard of operating in 'real time' so as to enable flexible modes of intervention while public health emergencies are occurring. In the previous form of international infectious disease control, international public health knowledge and the time of outbreak were asynchronous. WHO officials often did not know when outbreaks were occurring, or their knowledge occurred too late to prevent international transmission. Under emergency vigilance, public health knowledge is held to the standard of 'real time.' Real time or near-real time detection expands the range of possible public health responses to an international public health emergency.

There are many ways of partitioning time and many understandings of temporality, so the notion of 'real time' is at first puzzling, as the locution would seem prima facie to claim that some forms of time are more real than others, or perhaps that some forms of time are simply not real. Rather than wallow in this line of questioning, we prefer to treat 'real time' historically and begin by noting that it enters public health from computer science and communications. 'Real time' links two temporal orders with the intent of one modifying the other. 'Real-time computing' does not seek the fastest possible performance of a task; instead, it aims to optimize computer systems that fail or succeed in relation to a time at which a task needs to occur. This kind of computing is said to have 'real-time constraints,' that is, a deadline between the occurrence of an event and a response by the computing system.[4] The time of computing is articulated to the time of a phenomenon in which the computations are to intervene. Antilock brakes in automobiles, which must meet particular time constraints if they are to function effectively, is an example of real-time computing. Real-time computing involves the matching of two temporal orders, with cybernetic time adapting to the temporal organization present in the object of intervention.

Within the literature on mass communications 'real time' is not a technical concept but instead functions as a synonym for 'simultaneity' or 'speed.' In this sense, the antagonist of 'real time' is duration, or, more generally, this conception of 'real time' elides the significance of duration for processes of recognition and knowing.[5] Face-to-face communication is referred to as 'real time.' Satellite technology that allows images of events to be distributed to news outlets at close to the same time as these events are occurring is spoken of as operating in 'real time.' But for the most part, 'real time' is used in relation to technologically mediated communications that allow for what is called 'simultaneous communication,' that is, a pace of alternating communications similar to that of persons in a face-to-face speech situation.

A research participant clarified the public health sense of 'real time' used at WHO:

LW/EM: Everybody here talks about real time. And it's in the literature on outbreak detection. What does real time mean?

Research Participant: Real time means, for example in the SARS outbreak, that every day we were getting information, and some of that information was evidence, and some of that evidence was used to develop strategies or policies the next day. So real time means getting information at a time when something is happening, and then we take that information and we use it to develop policy or strategy or revise a policy and strategy at that time. That's a very important concept that moves forward in the International Health Regulations because they will be able in real time rather than in preestablished ways to recommend to countries how to stop the spread of an international event. (WHO Interview)

The research participant defines 'real time' in the communications sense as technologically mediated communication that enables knowledge of events to occur while the events are still in process. S/he emphasizes that for public health purposes real-time communications enable flexible governmental responses to the event as it is in process. Yet it might also be argued that real-time communications make possible not only flexible governmental responses, but also asymmetrical power relations as governance may increasingly know about and direct action in disparate local places, displacing the forms of local decision making that obtained under slower communications.

D) Public Health Emergencies and Security

Between the 1996 vision of a world on alert and the IHR (2005), a change had occurred. The world on alert had been securitized. Whereas the target of the world on alert, and indeed all prior international health law, had been communicable disease, the target of the IHR (2005) is international public health emergencies that include but extend beyond infectious disease. The concept of international public health emergency has been interpreted by WHO (2007: 17–33) to encompass foodborne illness; chemical, environmental, natural, nuclear and radiological disasters; and industrial accidents. International public health emergencies may be intentionally or unintentionally caused; they include the public health aspects of chemical, biological and radiological weapons use.

After the passage of the IHR (2005), WHO interestingly began to conceptualize international public health emergencies as matters of security. The Division of Emerging and Other Communicable Diseases that was constituted at WHO in October 1995 and later renamed Communicable Diseases in 1998 was reorganized and given a new title in 2008: the Health Security and Environment Cluster. It would no longer suffice to denominate the unit in terms of communicable diseases after the passage of the IHR (2005) had expanded action from infectious diseases to public health emergencies. "Communicable disease(s)" does not appear anywhere on the 2008 organizational chart for WHO headquarters.[6] This is not to say that communicable disease prevention and control has been eliminated in WHO programming, as 2008 WHO headquarters' structure includes the divisions of HIV/AIDS, TB, Malaria and Neglected Tropical Diseases and, in any case, organizational practices can't be read off organizational charts. But it is clear that it made little sense to formulate public health action that deals with international public health emergencies in terms of infectious disease control. Communicable disease control has been encompassed within public health security.

Yet what 'health security and environment' might mean is not obvious, as 'security' is widely used today and has many meanings. In the 2007 World Health Report, *A Safer Future: Global Public Health Security in the 21st Century*, global public health security is conceptualized as "the activities required, both proactive and reactive, to minimize vulnerability to acute public health events that endanger the collective health of populations living across geographical regions and international boundaries" (WHO 2007: 5). *A Safer Future* (WHO 2007: 17) links public health security to the expanded scope of international public health given under the IHR (2005). The concepts of public health security, public health events, and international public health emergency act in tandem to displace the previous concepts of communicable disease control and communicable disease, incorporating these within security.

Health security marks the articulation of global public health with international security. Since the seventeenth century, international security has concerned the relations across sovereign states, particularly war and peace together with the international treaties and agencies that structure relations among states. International security treaties such as the Biological and Toxin Weapons Convention and the Chemical Weapons Convention have historically been separate from international health law. Verifying international weapons incidents and dealing with their immediate impact on human health was a matter for international security, not international public health agencies. Of course, WHO, like many parts of the UN system, has a history of programming related to 'human security', a term that first gained currency after the publication of the 1994 Human Development report (United Nations Development Programme 1994). However, global health security, with its focus on transborder, acute, population health emergencies differs from human security which aims to provide the conditions for human health through practices that provide jobs, address hunger, increase welfare, reduce political oppression and social conflict, and deal with environmental hazards.

When emergency vigilance was being formed in the mid-to-late 1990s, it coincided with the invention of civilian biodefense, that is, the protection of civilian populations against bioweaspons use, not as previously solely military personnel in the field (Wright 2004), The growth of civilian bio-defense was also associated with the protection of national populations against EID, which then had the potential effect of making civilian infectious disease control relevant to biodefense. The 1990s were thus characterized by the growth of biosecurity thought and practice that sought to protect national and international security against harm from bioweapons and infectious diseases, The relation of the global emergency vigilance apparatus to biosecurity was thus a continuing question.

The association of bioweapons with infectious disease in the biosecurity concept links what had formerly been institutionally separate: public health and national and international security. As David Fidler and Lawrence Gostin (Fidler & Gostin 2008: 9) have observed, public health and security have historically been distinct policy areas both nationally and internationally. Our research shows that the integration of public health with biosecurity began as early as the first years of the 1990s in discussions about the need to create new techniques of infectious disease surveillance that would detect both intentionally caused and naturally occurring outbreaks of infectious disease. The formation of biosecurity as a policy domain thus occurred earlier than the intentional spread of anthrax in the USA during 2001 as some (Cooper 2006) have assumed. Since the mid-1990s biosecurity projects in global biopolitics have had a double object: bioweapons and the containment of EID.

In international public health the discussion of the need for better EID surveillance was conceptually coordinated with bioweapons surveillance, and both were integrated into the functioning of early warning outbreak detection. As discussed in Chapter 3, a series of papers about the need for improved global epidemiological surveillance and field investigations of biological and chemical warfare appeared in the journal *Politics and the Life Sciences* during 1992, with Stephen Morse (1992; member, Federation of American Scientists' Working Group on Biological and Toxin Weapons Verification and later [1994–2000] program manager for Biodefense at the Defense Advanced Research Projects Agency [DARPA], U.S. Department of Defense), Barbara Hatch Rosenberg (1992; coordinator, Federation of American Scientists' Biological and Toxin Weapons Verification Working Group), and Jack Woodall (1992; WHO, Geneva), all of whom were later active in the founding of ProMED-mail, responding to papers by Mark Wheelis (1992; University of California, Davis) and Peter Barss (1992; Montreal General Hospital and McGill University). Hatch Rosenberg and Woodall replied to Wheelis's article and argued that his proposal for a global epidemiological surveillance network needed to be primarily motivated in terms of communicable disease prevention and control, with bioweapons detection as a secondary goal. Morse (1992: 29) suggested that surveillance and field investigations should include all unexpected outbreaks: "A global capacity for recognizing and responding to unexpected outbreaks of disease, by allowing the early identification and control of disease outbreaks, would simultaneously buttress defenses against both diseases and CBTW [chemical, biological, and toxin weapons]." These articles by some of the most significant figures in the establishment of ProMED-mail show that in the early 1990s online early warning outbreak detection was being conceptualized as a technique bridging public health and security.

The securitizing of global emergency vigilance continued in the IHR (2005). For the first time in the history of international health law, "the IHR 2005 applies to public health events that may involve the intentional use of biological agents or that may stem from illicit activities involving biological agents" (Fidler & Gostin 2008: 138). The infectious disease lists found in international health law during the late 19th and 20th centuries required mandatory report solely for diseases that were presumed to be "naturally occurring." Deliberate use of bioweapons was prohibited under treaties such as the Geneva Protocol (1925) that were not part of international health law (Fidler & Gostin 2008: 1). The legal concepts of public health event, public health risk, and public health emergency of international concern found in the IHR (2005) are novel in a number of ways, one of which is that they may be applied to both naturally occurring and intentionally caused emergencies, including bioweapons use.

The securitizing of emergency vigilance initiates a form of watchfulness over both naturally occurring infectious diseases and acts that violate international treaties, reading each as threats to social and political order detectable by the same public health methods. Whereas the alert and risk apparatuses discussed by Chateauraynaud and Torny (1999) protect individual and collective bodies against damage from legally authorized industries such as nuclear power and meat, the IHR (2005) seeks to protect WHO country members and the international system against the public health effects related to the deliberate or accidental release of pathogens and other weapons.

Integrating biosecurity and other forms of security concern into emergency vigilance posed a continuing series of boundary problems for WHO, which as an inter-state organization is required to maintain diplomatic neutrality with respect to its member states. Extending WHO's mandate to public health emergencies potentially included detecting and responding to to chemical, biological, radiological, and nuclear incidents. This raised questions as to what WHO's role should be under these conditions in relation to other agencies in the UN system, to external agencies with which WHO collaborates, and to WHO standards-setting practices. The final process of revising the IHR (2005) occurred under the impetus of SARS, but also in a context influenced by the deliberate spread of anthrax in the USA during 2001. Under pressure to respond to bioweapons threats, WHO consistently distinguished between public health issues that fell within its mandate and non-public health issues for which other UN and international agencies were responsible. The WHO Programme for Preparedness for Deliberate Epidemics was established under World Health Assembly Resolution 55.16 in May 2002. Its 2004–2005 annual programme stressed that disarmament and nonproliferation were matters for the Biological Weapons Convention rather than WHO: "The primary emphasis of WHO's work on deliberately caused diseases is on public health preparedness and response to the deliberate use of biological agents that affect health" (WHO 2004: 114). One of our WHO research participants emphasized that there is a clear line of report for WHO if, when in the field, an emergency should turn out to have been deliberately caused. Under these circumstances WHO would report to the UN Security Council, which would then take over the investigation, leaving WHO to focus its field response on public health (WHO Interview).

The boundary between WHO and national security came up in relation to GPHIN. After the 2003 SARS outbreak, the U.S. Armed Forces Medical Intelligence Center became a client of GPHIN. This challenged the relationship between GPHIN and WHO, its collaborating partner, on the grounds that WHO could not be associated with intelligence organizations. For this and other reasons, GPHIN and WHO redefined their relation, and WHO became a client of GPHIN. A further instance of the boundary work WHO did in the process of defining its relation to security occurred in the extension of WHO laboratory standards for biosafety (which ensure against unintended or accidental exposure to pathogens or toxins) to include biosecurity (which protects against the intentional harm from pathogens or toxins) (WHO 2006; Atlas & Reppy 2005).

After full drafts of the IHR became available in 2004–2005, the boundary between what should and what should not fall within WHO's public health mandate was debated between North and South. The working drafts of the IHR required States Parties to "provide WHO with all relevant public health information, materials and samples" (Fidler 2005: 356) if a member state had evidence to show that a chemical, biological or radiological weapon had been intentionally released in its territory. The USA and its allies supported this provision (called Article 45 in the September 2004 and January 2005 drafts, Article 41 in the January 2004 draft) as it would have given access to valuable intelligence information otherwise unobtainable. In December 2004 the report of the UN Secretary-General's High Level Panel on Threats, Challenges and Change recommended that WHO advise the UN Security Council of disease outbreaks possibly caused by deliberate chemical, biological, and radiological weapons use. This report fueled political opposition to Article

45. In January 2005, the governments of Argentina, Bolivia, Brazil, Chile, Columbia, Ecuador, Peru, Uruguay and Venezuela jointly issued the Montevideo Document, which argued that there was no cause for specific language in the IHR to deal with suspected or deliberate release of chemical, biological or radiological agents since, if such releases were to become an international public health risk, they would be adequately addressed under other provisions of the IHR (Fidler 2005: 365, n. 218). Andrew Kelle's interview research with national delegates who had participated in the rounds of negotiations prior to the passing of the IHR in May 2005 showed that WHO country members from the global South "mostly from the Southeast Asia and eastern Mediterranean regional group, were led in their rejection [of Article 45] by Pakistani and Iranian delegates" (Kelle 2007: 227). The proposal that chemical, biological, radiological and nuclear incidents be made notifiable under the IHR was also turned down (ibid). As a result of the interventions by WHO's country members from the global South and negotiations with collaborating partners, WHO's security mandate under the IHR was restricted to organizing public health responses to chemical, biological, radiological, and nuclear incidents and to assisting international preparedness and response programmes.

WHO was given an international security mandate under the IHR (2005). It became the premier organization dealing with the public health aspects of international disasters, deliberately and non-deliberately caused. Global public health had been securitized, but the meaning of security had been confined to the alleviation of acute, population-based, public health events.

*   *   *

We have argued that global emergency vigilance represents an epistemological shift in international communicable disease control as it existed at WHO prior to 1995. The transformation in knowledge involved a new and expansive conceptualization of the target of public health action as international public health emergencies, the rising significance of surface knowledge and its coordination with depth knowledge, a real-time temporal standard, and the securitizing of the vigilance apparatus.

The epistemological shift was, as we discussed in Chapter 2, driven by the political demand for new forms of global public health governance. For many in the global North and international public health, this represented an opportunity to revitalize public health, but the revitalization would occur in ways that reduced the political question to worst-case scenarios and biosecurity. The utopian horizon of public health after World War II, health as well-being, and the participatory social democratic vision of the Health for All strategy of the 1970s and 1980s had been transformed into an horizon of constant danger.

WHO as a Suprasovereign Power

The realization of emergency vigilance as a governance form required the emancipation of epidemiological knowledge from sovereign power.

Emergency vigilance marks the formation of a new political level in bio-politics, a biopolitical level beyond that of sovereign states. With the passage of the IHR (2005), WHO became a limited global power, authorized to legally know about and announce international public health emergencies, if necessary without the cooperation of the sovereign states that are its country members. The IHR (2005) transformed the power/knowledge relations for international public health by authorizing WHO to have powers of suprasovereign knowledge and political speech.

We use governance in the broad Foucauldian sense (discussed previously) to mean the conduct of conduct: the schemes devised by authorities for the right disposition of humans, nonhuman species, and things. A governance strategy for global emergency vigilance was projected in the WHO strategic planning document Emerging and Other Communicable Disease (WHO 1996), which clearly defined a series of governance goals for "a world on alert" (WHO 1996: n.p.). Public health vision in a world on alert is oriented to rapid national and international surveillance, information exchange, preparedness, and response. The world on alert has a single overarching objective: the containment of international communicable disease outbreaks. Containment at the global level requires coordinated action to prevent disease transmission into a region or regions where a disease has been eradicated from regions in which it is endemic. A second sense of containment refers to preventing transmission of communicable disease beyond a locus, in this case across international boundaries.

As we outlined more fully in Chapter 3, the world on alert as a governance strategy took rapid institutional form at WHO between 1995 and 2000. The first of the multinational global response teams was assembled in 1995 to help with the Ebola outbreak in Kikwit, Zaire. In October 1995 the Division of Emerging and other Communicable Diseases Surveillance and Control was established, followed by GOARN officially in 2000, but which had been in formation from 1997. GPHIN, the early warning outbreak alert and detection system, became operational and began work with WHO in 1998. Between 1998 and 2000 WHO developed the Outbreak Verification Team as a social and political solution to aligning unofficial information with sovereign confirmation of epidemiological information.

During the period between 1998 and 2003 WHO experimented with the governance apparatus for global emergency vigilance. Some aspects of this experimentation were, as David Fidler (2004b: 143) has emphasized, in contravention of then-existing international public health law, but were authorized under a series of resolutions passed by the World Health Assembly. These included the two 1995 resolutions (discussed in Chapter 2) that called for the revision of the IHR (1969) (WHA48.7, Revision and Updating of the International Health Regulations (World Health Assembly 1995a)) and fundamental changes to WHO's system of communicable disease control (WHA 48.13, Communicable disease prevention and control: new, emerging and re-emerging infectious diseases (World Health Assembly 1995b)). These resolutions indicated a willingness of WHO members to change international health law, but public health practices routinely outstripped legal mandate during the period 1998–2003. By way of example, when during the SARS outbreak WHO issued its first global alert on March 12, 2003, it did not have the legal mandate to do so until May 2003 through a resolution of the World Health Assembly (Fidler 2004b: 143).

The experimentation between 1998 and 2003 that created a governance apparatus for global emergency vigilance contravened international health law. WHO effectively treated WHA48.7, Revision and Updating of the International Health Regulations, as though it suspended the IHR (1969), although the Regulations still remained in force. One might say that WHO acted in anticipation of a law that was in formation, a future law. It would be incorrect, however, to interpret this period as a state of exception, a concept introduced by the political philosopher Carl Schmitt to theorize sovereignty. Schmitt (1922/1985) argued that sovereignty consists of more than the power to break or rescind particular laws. The sovereign may suspend law as such, in particular the law of the constitution. In the suspension of the normal juridical order, the sovereign declares the state of exception. The WHO Constitution was not suspended at the turn of the 21st century. The experimentation simply broke the law, although it was done publicly and with the full knowledge of WHO member countries.

Instead of extending the concept, state of exception, without limit after the current fashion, it is more productive to theorize with precision spaces that border on it and differentiate their dangers. The space considered here may be termed 'pure governance,' a condition that arises when the political suffers governance to invent new forms of governance beyond law in the political promise of new law. Pure governance is the violation of a law that none seek to apply, an experimental space between past and future right. One danger of pure governance is that new legislation might never occur, in which case governance might proceed indefinitely. Pure governance is one of the many challenges to international politics and law in our present, as international political institutions are only weakly formed and the rule of law in the area of global biosecurity poorly established (Fidler & Gostin 2008: 13–15) while the invention of governance proceeds apace. The existence of pure governance in international health law and politics is one reason to think carefully about the question of the political in excess of the governmental, a question we consider shortly.

The pure governance apparatus for emergency vigilance challenged the relation that had been established in the second half of the 20th century between official and unofficial information about outbreak. During those decades—what we termed the postcolonial period in international public health—the unofficial outbreak information that flowed into WHO was not a 'knowledge of record' that could be given to WHO's country members, nor could it be publicly announced, a principle that was tested when the WHO secretariat announced the 1970 cholera outbreak in Guinea without sovereign consent (see Chapter 3 for discussion). Despite the fact that the ISR (1951) and the IHR (1969) had specific language that required WHO's sovereign members to report cases of notifiable diseases, noncompliance was routine. International health law passed by the World Health Assembly notoriously suffered from what has been called the 'sovereignty problem' in international law as the ISR (1951) and the IHR (1969) lacked sanctions for noncompliance. Under these conditions state sovereignty trumped international health governance when conflict arose regarding reporting. But during the pure governance phase of emergency vigilance the detection of actual, emerging, and potential international public health events occurred in real time with unofficial, transnationalized data sources—detection that was being used in ways that clearly transcended international law, as did WHO's public announcements made on the basis of this information.

The International Health Regulations (2005) effected a fundamental displacement of the sovereignty problem in international public health law by authorizing WHO to collect unofficial epidemiological information, to announce global alerts without sovereign consent if urgently necessary, and to issue travel advisories and other communications during emergencies. The sovereign states that are members of WHO are given the obligation of replying to WHO requests for outbreak verification within 24 hours. In the event the sovereign member should not collaborate with WHO's requests for information, WHO may share unofficial information with its other country members "when justified by the magnitude of public health risk" (IHR 2005: Art. 10). WHO was granted the power of announcing emergencies "to the public" without the cooperation of the affected sovereign under conditions when the emergency "has already become publicly available and there is a need for the dissemination of authoritative and independent information" (IHR 2005: Art. 11). The IHR (2005) gave WHO powers it did not formerly have, what one member of the U.S. CDC has hyperbolically called "'police' powers for controlling outbreaks that put it above national governments" (Piller as cited in Fidler 2004b: 143). The IHR (2005) conferred on WHO powers beyond those of its sovereign members, but these powers do not include the right of crossing into or otherwise intervening in the territories of its members without sovereign consent.

The new powers granted to WHO in the IHR (2005) brought the pure governance system of emergency vigilance within international health law. In granting WHO the power to have a knowledge of record based on unofficial sources, WHO was given an informal power of sanction, although the economic and political effects associated with the announcement of international public health emergencies are not the work of WHO, but rather a reaction to it. The IHR (2005) is thus unlike the IHR (1969) in being more than a political norm of international cooperation systematically violated in practice; WHO is permitted at the level of law to have unofficial knowledge about international public health events and the power to declare an emergency without sovereign consent. Sovereign states cooperate with WHO in anticipation of these powers over and above the resources such as vaccines and pharmaceuticals that WHO is able to provide. Thus under the IHR (2005) WHO attains a series of suprasovereign powers. In this manner another level of political power was distinguished from sovereignty in global biopolitics. We have called this level suprasovereign to indicate a level of power beyond the sovereign.

Emergency vigilance thus represents an epistemological shift that was first realized in an experimental space of pure governance and subsequently given the form of juridical right. The general movement across law, governance, and the political may be characterized as the emancipation of epidemiological knowledge from sovereign power. In the IHR (2005) the sovereign states that are the members of WHO agreed to legally authorize the ability of the WHO governance apparatus to know about public health emergencies and, where the governance apparatus judges necessary, to announce them in the absence of sovereign collaboration. This is what we mean by the emancipation of knowledge from sovereignty. The knowledge practices that the World Health Assembly emancipated are institutionally located, not in the legislature or the executive of WHO, but in WHO governance bodies, in particular the WHO Secretariat (the day-to-day WHO staff in Geneva concerned with the governance of international health) and GOARN, the WHO collaborative network. The ultimate power of announcing a public health emergency to the global media, thereby potentially creating a global media event along the lines of that which happened in the SARS outbreak, is a suprasovereign speech act that vests with WHO governance.

Let us put the constitution of WHO as a suprasovereign power in a broader historical context. In passing the IHR (2005), the World Health Assembly revised the political conception of the extraterritorial interests of sovereign states with respect to the common threat of infectious diseases. In the mid-17th century sovereignty was territorialized at the Peace of Westphalia as a European system of distinct states, each having absolute power internally, although externally existing in a state of nature with respect to each other, that is, without law or a common polity. Sovereign states nonetheless had interests beyond their own territories, notably in their colonial possessions, but also in who and what crossed their borders. From the late 19th century certain infectious diseases such as plague and cholera were recognized as common threats; these threats were defined in international health law through lists of named infectious diseases. The specifics about the resources to be allocated to international infectious disease control and what questions sovereign powers should be asked and should not be asked about infectious diseases were in part scientific questions, but they were also political questions about who rules and in whose interests. During the period of Euro-American colonization epidemiological intelligence was taken from colonies, which were not recognized as sovereign, by colonial powers. As the Euro-American colonies became independent states from the late 1940s to the 1960s, they asserted sovereign control over epidemiological communications. In the second half of the 20th century, epidemiological information remained firmly under ultimate sovereign control. With the ascendance of global emergency vigilance, consolidated at law in the IHR (2005), knowledge pertinent to international public health emergencies was freed from ultimate sovereign control as the

World Health Assembly redefined the common extraterritorial health threat to be of such an order that it warranted a diminishment of sovereign power.

Although we have argued that WHO has become a suprasovereign power in the area of public health emergencies of international concern, we do not wish to be mistaken for arguing that the sovereign level of power has somehow been abolished or transcended. In the recent 'country compact' model of development assistance for health, the International Health Partnership negotiates with sovereign states for multiyear health programming (see Chapter 2). This model has arisen in the context of uncoordinated, short-term development assistance for health by multiple donors that led countries in the global South to protest losing control of their health care systems. What the sovereign level of power suffers as a political loss to the suprasovereign level in global emergency vigilance may be regained and consolidated elsewhere.

The degree to which public health knowledge of events has been emancipated from sovereignty will clearly be tested in future. The first WHO advisory against nonessential travel to Toronto, Beijing, and Shanxi Province (China) announced on April 23, 2003 was immediately resisted by Health Canada (Whaley & Mansoor 2006: 33, 35) and became the focus of a political struggle on the part of Canadian politicians to have it withdrawn, which the WHO did on April 30, 2003. How the United States of America, that most sovereign of sovereign states,[7] would react to equivalent uses against itself of WHO powers under the IHR (2005) is yet to be known. Such a test of the effective suprasovereign powers of WHO would partially repeat the scenario of the 1970 cholera outbreak that the Republic of Guinea refused to report and which was announced by the WHO governance apparatus (see Chapter 3, p. 74–75). That announcement created a division in WHO between its governance section, which includes the Secretariat, and the World Health Assembly, the center of political power at WHO. If a similar situation were to happen under the IHR (2005) but involved the EU or the USA, WHO's political and governance centers might again enter into conflict, with results unknown at the present time.

In their much-read book *Empire*, Michael Hardt and Antonio Negri (2000: 4) argued that the UN has served as a "hinge in the genealogy from international to global juridical structures." The UN becomes effective, they write, "only insofar as it transfers sovereign right into a real *supranational* center" (Hardt & Negri 2000: 5; their emphasis). Their analysis applies well to the role that WHO as a UN agency has played in the passage from international infectious disease control to a new juridical order in global public health. For WHO to fulfill its constitutional mandate in international communicable disease control required the emancipation of epidemiological knowledge about international public health events and emergencies from sovereign control in the second half of the 20th century and its transference to WHO as a supranational center.

Hardt and Negri propose empire—which they call "imperial sovereignty"—as the current logic of world order beyond national sovereignty. Empire, they write, is characterized by (1) rule without spatial/political boundaries, (2) rule without historical/temporal boundaries related to an origin in conquest, and (3) rule that attempts to regulate all social and life processes. With respect to spatial boundaries, Hardt and Negri (2000: xiv–xv) argue that empire intervenes by suspending all law (instituting a state of exception) and sends in the military anywhere/everywhere on humanitarian or other universal/ethical grounds. Yet empire, whose content is capital, cannot stabilize a normative system of juridical and political right for its social and economic relations (Hardt & Negri 2000: 394) due to the resistance of the multitude who, in a sudden dialectical reversal, constitute themselves as the new global proletariat.

Contemporary world order lacks the uniformity that Hardt and Negri theorize; recognizing and theorizing its unevenness and patchiness is an alternative writing strategy to producing universal histories such as theirs. Our comments here do not model all world order on WHO's form of suprasovereignty so much as insist that WHO is part of world order and that it does not conform to imperial sovereignty. The characteristic features of imperial sovereignty fit the case of global emergency vigilance rather badly. WHO has neither the juridical right nor the substantive capacity to invade the territories of its sovereign members; it has no military or police powers. WHO must have sovereign consent before a response team crosses the territorial boundaries of a sovereign state. WHO has suprasovereign powers of knowledge and speech, but its material, embodied powers do not extend limitlessly in space. Although epidemiological information about international public health events is no longer wholly under sovereign control (with an ongoing countervailing struggle by some nation-states), at the level of intervention, whether with vaccines or response teams, global emergency vigilance is rule within spatial/political boundaries. As to its historical sense, WHO, like most medical organizations, has a well-honed interest in producing monumental histories that attest to its accomplishments, dating its founding to that of the UN system at the end of World War II. Nonetheless, global emergency vigilance was constituted outside the system of juridical right under conditions we have called pure governance. But this state of pure governance is not equivalent to the permanent state of exception that Hardt and Negri argue characterizes empire because global emergency vigilance was eventually given juridical form in the period between 2003 and 2005. Pure governance needs to be examined and theorized in its specificity rather than collapsed into the state of exception, a concept that is overextended by Hardt and Negri.

Although our work about global emergency vigilance has been framed in relation to biopolitics, we have not followed Hardt and Negri's identification of biopolitics with the forces of production and social reproduction that attempt to regulate all social and life processes.[8] As a biopolitical strategy, global emergency vigilance was born at the moment the expansionist, modernist fantasy of regulating all social and life processes failed, fear of infectious disease outbreaks spread once more in the global North, and a policy of containment supplemented by humanitarian assistance was implemented.

Conceptualizing the Political in Global Biopolitics

Global emergency vigilance is in one sense a case study of the world order that is being constituted beyond the political relations that had characterized sovereignty and its system of interstate relations. As the previous section of this chapter argued, another level of political power has been juridically instituted to deal with international public health emergencies. In turn, this suprasovereign political level has effects on and reconstructs the sovereign level of power in public health. We now turn to the questions of whether suprasovereign power is to be identified with governance and, more generally, how to conceptualize the political. To this point we have presupposed a division between governance and the political rather than argued for it. The distinction drawn here between governance and the political is at variance with expansive meanings given to governance in global health policy (Aginam 2005b; Hein, Bartsch, & Kohlmorgen 2007; Lee 2003; Zacher 2008) and the Foucauldian literature (Dean 2007; Larner & Walters 2004a; O'Malley, Weir, & Shearing 1997; Rose 1999; Rose, O'Malley, & Valverde 2006; Weir 1996). Recent Foucauldian-influenced anthropological collections on biopolitics (Ong & Collier 2005; Inda 2005) expand the term governance such that it becomes coterminous with the political. However, emergency vigilance as a research site centrally poses the question of the relation between governance and the political on the terrain of biopolitics.

We wish to complicate the understanding of 'politics' in biopolitics, and argue first that the concept of the political is not equivalent to governance. Second, sovereignty is an historically specific form of the political, not a transhistorical term. The effect of these distinctions on the concept of global biopolitics is to enable a differentiated conception of contemporary biopolitics, with irreducible suprasovereign, sovereign, and governance levels articulated to each other. Our argument parallels Mitchell Dean's (2004) theorization of the nomos of the earth—the appropriation, partitioning, and cultivation of land—as distinct from and prior to governmentality, although we have not theorized the political through Schmitt's concept of nomos, turning instead to Lefort's conception of common fate and the symbolic. This theorization enables a conception of WHO as a suprasovereign power that is not reducible to the positive theory of law as explicit statements of recognized authorities backed by the power of sanction. Contemporary international health law is dominated by positive theories of law, partly due to the influence of David Fidler's important work. We provide here an alternative formulation.

The health policy and Foucauldian literatures have pursued what is in many ways a parallel trajectory in conflating governance with the political. A conceptual review of "global health governance" by Dodgson, Lee, and Drager (2002) carefully analyzes the meanings given to 'governance' in the international health policy literature. Their review was commissioned by WHO and jointly issued by WHO Geneva and the London School of Hygiene and Tropical Medicine (Dodgson, Lee, & Drager 2002): an authoritative institutional positioning. Dodgson, Lee, and Drager (2002: 6) define "health governance" as "the actions and means adopted by a society to organize itself in the promotion and protection of the health of its population."[9] In their account, 'government' differs from 'governance' in having formalized rules and procedures that are backed by formal authority and sanctions (ibid.). They place governance and government on a scale from the informal to the formal. Yet Dodgson, Lee, and Drager then categorize government as a particular form of governance with no clear justification made for governance as the dominant term; a third term would be logically required to name the scale. In any case, the result of these analytic moves is to encompass the political within governance. Similarly, the majority of Foucauldian scholars writing on government, with the exception of Dean (1999, 2004) and Dillon (1995), treat government, originally defined against sovereignty, as identical to the political (Singer & Weir 2006: 449–450).[10] By way of example, in Powers of Freedom, a comprehensive overview of Foucauldian work on governance by a much-respected scholar, Nikolas Rose (1999: 3, 15) suggests replacing the study of politics and the state with government.[11]

Foucault's own treatment of the relation between the political and what he called "governmentality" is situated in the context of his unsettled and inconsistent treatment of sovereignty (Singer & Weir 2006). He defines the specificity of governmentality as a new form of political reasoning that originated in 16th-century critiques of Machiavelli. In the early modern period the governmental form of reasoning turned its gaze away from the prince and towards the relations between people and mundane things in order to promote the wealth and health of political subjects (Foucault 2000a: 208). In some passages Foucault treats governmentality as displacing sovereignty: "The old power of death that symbolized sovereign power was now carefully supplanted by the administration of bodies and the calculated management of life" (Foucault 1976/1978: 139–140); "The more I have spoken about population, the more I have stopped saying 'sovereign'" (Foucault 2007: 76). Yet in other passages Foucault treated sovereignty as present in the 20th century, notably in his analysis of the biopolitics, particularly of the Holocaust (Foucault 1976/1978: 135–159; Foucault 2003: 258–261).

There is much at stake in refusing to reduce the political to governance/governmentality. In articles cowritten with Brian Singer (Singer & Weir 2006, 2008), Lorna Weir sought to trouble the Foucauldian identification of governance with the political and the resulting elision/minimization of sovereignty. Singer and Weir defended a stronger conception of sovereignty, one that did not disappear with the early modern 'absolute' monarchs. The democratic sovereign, by way of example, has been in existence since the second half of the 18th century (Singer & Weir 2008: 55–58); the communist and fascist sovereigns date to the 20th century. Without a conception of sovereign power it is not possible to theorize or diagnose the dangers of the state of exception, where law as such is suspended. Governmentality thrives in the state of exception, doing the bidding of the sovereign, without the sovereign's police and military powers being checked by law (Singer & Weir 2008: 58–63). Last, the reduction of the political to governance ignores at least half the significance of Machiavelli. Machiavelli's historical importance lies in theorizing the political as a relation between rulers and ruled with no ultimate solution (Singer & Weir 2008: 50–55). Thus, rather than using governance to erase sovereignty, or the reverse, sovereignty and governmentality are intelligible only by reference to each other, with the many projects of governance to make better economies, stronger soldiers, longer-lived populations, and so forth having sovereign power as their condition of existence.

The question arises as to whether the sovereignty concept should be used to characterize the political forms that are presently in formation beyond the level of the sovereign state. Many would prefer to use sovereignty in an expansive, transhistorical sense, for instance Agamben (1998), who locates its formation in ancient Rome and treats its principles as alive in contemporary biopolitics, particularly in proliferating states of exception. Hardt and Negri (2000: 93–113, 183–204) periodize sovereignty into two successive phases: modern sovereignty of the nation-state (from roughly the 16th century to the mid-20th century) and the imperial sovereignty of our present, with its distinctive form of imperial biopolitics. Our own preference is to retain the historical specificity of sovereignty and resist identifying it with the political as such.

We understand sovereignty as the form in which the political was imagined and given institutional form from roughly the 16th century (although its intellectual lineage extends from the 14th; see Bartelson 1995: 101–107) into the 20th century. It was only in the late medieval period that sovereignty appeared as a locution, one that came to be borne during the 17th century by a determinate institutional form, the territorially based nation-state. As Carl Schmitt (Ojakangas 2006: 172–173) argued, early modern sovereignty was characterized by the subordination of disparate medieval legal systems—feudal, ecclesiastical, estate, and territorial—to the administration, judiciary, and legislation of the territorial ruler. Sovereignty also marked the end of the civil wars of religion in Europe, as the religion of the territory was determined by its sovereign rather than by the Pope. Sovereignty applied over a territory absolutely. In relation to each other, sovereigns had impermeable territorial boundaries. The beginnings of international law took the form of relations between European states, with their colonies subject to European sovereignty and its civilizing mission (Anghie 2007: 3–7). Once the substance of sovereignty is conceptualized in this specific historical sense, which we have done no more than gloss over here, sovereignty cannot be equated with a transhistorical conception of the political. Nor can the concept of sovereignty and its associated form of world order be applied in any obvious sense to the international relations that began to be constituted in the 20th century from the period of the League of Nations, international relations that traversed the previously impermeable boundaries of sovereign power (Schmitt 1932/1996: 55–56). The organizing principles of world order that Schmitt termed the *jus publicum Europaeum* (European public law) have been at least partially displaced by new understandings of warfare over the course of the 20th and early 21st centuries (Schmitt 1932/1996: chap. 4, "Transformation of the Meaning of War"; Hardt & Negri 2000: 34–38), and both the law of property and the criminal law are no longer solely sovereign matters that fall within national jurisdiction.

We might have elected, as did Hardt and Negri, to theorize emergency vigilance in global biopolitics through the concept of sovereignty, but such a move would have required a conception of sovereignty that breaks with the defining characteristics of sovereignty for roughly the past 4 centuries. Instead, and for this reason, we have not used the sovereignty concept to theorize the political beyond governance in global biopolitics, preferring the provisional term of suprasovereign, that is, above the sovereign.

The question then arises as to how the political in global biopolitics is to be theorized. Following a long tradition in political philosophy, we treat the political as a relation established between human beings in response to "the question on which their common fate depends" (Lefort 1988: 49). There is, we remark, nothing prima facie good or wise in the ways common fates are imagined—although whatever the fate chosen, a division between the political 'us' and the 'non-us' is necessarily constituted. The political is instituted symbolically as a "space that can, despite its internal heterogeneity, perceive itself in its entirety" (Lefort 1988: 3). The institution of the political through the symbolic formation of a common fate creates a joint world rendered intelligible through particular meanings given to the just and the unjust, the permitted and the forbidden, the real and the unreal (Lefort 1988: 12). Lefort's theorization of the political differs from Schmitt's (1932/1996) in its emphasis on solidarity and intelligibility rather than the friend/enemy distinction. In so doing, Lefort's conception of the political addresses the constitution of political recognition and collectivity rather than presupposing it, a weakness in Schmitt's work.

The formation of the political is accomplished through a form of discourse that is characteristic of neither science nor governance: the symbolic. The symbolic combines words and things, that is, representation and presentation, in a particular way. Presentation refers to how things are made available for knowledge. Representation concerns how things, once rendered present, are given for a second time in speech, or writing, or song, or drawings—any signifying practice. Presentation and representation may take many different forms, which in turn combine in various ways. In the symbolic, representation manifests presentation (Singer & Weir 2006: 453–454; Weir 2008). Although things may exist prior to their representation in the symbolic, they are only made accessible to humans when they are represented. Politics, law, and religion are forms of the symbolic found in our present. Juridical law does not name a world of things that exists before the law is passed; rather, in law representation forms presentation. In the political symbolic, the sovereign is formed in representation; the people as democratic sovereign do not exist as a thing prior to representation in political speech. The symbolic gives sense, coherence, and order to what is represented; it has a normative horizon of world making. At another and more abstract level, differing symbolic forms such as law and the political enter into relation with each other in what Lefort (1986; 1988) has called the "symbolic regime." The relations between law, the political, and knowledge in global emergency vigilance are examined here, but this analysis borders on without crossing over into theorizing a global symbolic regime, as this does not presently exist.

Although Lefort's work has for the most part dealt with theorizing the political at the level of national sovereignty, his conception of the political as the symbolic recognition of a common fate can be applied to the political in global public health. In the 1946 WHO Constitution (ratified in 1948), health is the common fate that gives rise to WHO as a political body: "The objective of the World Health Organization (hereinafter called the Organization) shall be the attainment by all peoples of the highest possible level of health" (WHO 1946: Art. 1). The preamble to the WHO Constitution famously conceptualized health capaciously: "Health is a state of complete physical, mental and social well-being and not merely the absence of disease or infirmity" (WHO 1946). The excess of health over illness given in the term "well-being" was unprecedented in prior international health agreements, as was the identification of health as a fundamental right (Fantini 1993: 450). As a symbolic construct of international law, health as "well-being" forms a utopia that simultaneously aspires to achieve complete well-being and the absence of disease for all the peoples of the world: a politically established horizon of public health governance.

WHO did not exist prior to the law that enacted it; representation here constitutes presentation, that is, the formation of WHO was a symbolic act. The common fate that WHO was formed to address conferred an (expansively) coherent objective on WHO. In order to enhance the political objective of health, the Constitution of the World Health Organization lays out a broad programme of public functions that include medical and scientific research, governance, education for health and the formation of "public opinion," and political work such as the promotion of conventions and agreements dealing with health (WHO 1946: Art. 2). The symbolic horizon of WHO was formed after World War II in a moment of optimism about the possibility of what might be called 'permanent health.' One example of this is WHO's constitutional functions "to stimulate and advance work to eradicate epidemic, endemic and other diseases" (WHO 1946: Art. 2). The goal is not to contain the transmission of disease and treat the ill, but to eradicate diseases, as indeed occurred with smallpox for a brief moment in the last decades of the 20th century.

The World Health Assembly, a name that implies a deliberative and legislative body rather than a governance one, is the center of political power at WHO, a representative body composed of three delegates from each of the sovereign states that are WHO members. The health law passed by the World Health Assembly is shaped by what these sovereign Member States perceive to be their common fate with respect to health and what they need to know, singly and collectively, to deal with this common fate. The EID concept, for instance, was initially used to redefine what the USA and its allies in the global North needed to know about infectious disease outbreaks in order to protect their citizens against disease transmission. Under pressure from its members in the global North, the World Health Assembly accepted in 1995 that the common threat from infectious diseases had changed and that both WHO and its members needed to know much more about outbreaks, and to know faster and earlier.

The World Health Assembly, although a delegated assembly rather than a democratic body established by the people, nonetheless establishes a political scene in which divisions enter into debate. WHO's sovereign members and regional power blocs debate the formation of health law in terms that exceed the positive conception of law, which remains content with an understanding of law as that which has the power of sanction and is the output of a legally constituted body. The World Health Assembly debates the law in terms of justice across its political divisions, of which there are many: North and South, rich and poor, the USA and other powers, differences across WHO's six world regions, and so forth.

In the 1946 WHO Constitution, WHO was given many governance functions, among them collaboration with the UN and other governmental and professional groups, promotion of better teaching standards, and the development of international standards for pharmaceuticals as well as international nomenclature for diseases (WHO 1946: Art. 2). In communicable disease control WHO has a public health mandate that seeks to protect health on a population basis rather than on an individual basis. Many aspects of global emergency vigilance involved the formation of governance concepts and practices such as early warning detection, outbreak alerts, and global response teams. Emergency vigilance also involved the creation of institutional forms that included the WHO Division of Emerging and other Communicable Diseases Surveillance and Control (discussed in Chapter 2), Epidemic and Pandemic Alert and Response in the later Division of Health Security and Environment, GOARN, and GPHIN.

We note that the governance infrastructure of global emergency vigilance does not have robust funding, even though it represents an epistemological shift in public health and the formation of WHO as a suprasovereign power. Emergency vigilance is brilliance on a small budget. WHO supplies GOARN with a small administrative staff that includes an operational support team, a project manager, and assistance for a steering committee (Hitchcock et al. 2007: 218). Although most members cover their own costs of participation, there is no budget for GOARN work provided by WHO, and field responses must be funded by staff through fundraising outside WHO each time a response occurs (Chu 2005). The U.S.-based Nuclear Fund Initiative provided GOARN with the WHO-NTI Global Emergency Response Fund, a revolving fund of US$500,000 that may be allocated to immediate mobilization of response teams with the provision that the expenditures are later reimbursed (Hitchcock et al. 2007: 218). In an October 2006 interview, a WHO research participant reported the total biennial budget of Epidemic and Pandemic Alert and Response as US$220 million, but the effective budget allocated by WHO was US$11 million, that is, 5% of the biennial budget came from WHO's regular budget. The remainder of the budget was raised directly from donors. WHO research participants expressed frustration that much of their work time was spent raising US$2 million per week (WHO Interview).

Governance bridges fact and norm. It does not just seek to represent things, but also tries to make normative interventions to effect the right disposition of persons and things so that persons, populations, and polities may become healthy and wealthy. Governance thus has a symbolic axis that seeks through representation to render things present (Singer & Weir 2006: 457; Weir 2008: 377–378). In the case of WHO, the governance practice of rendering health present as well-being does not simply document illness neutrally, but also tries to create the conditions for health to occur. Governance practices the normative in the name of the empirical and practices the empirical in the name of the normative. The political as a symbolic knowledge and governance as a practice that combines both symbolic and empirical knowledge are thus not identical. The political symbolic of WHO creates a common world from deliberations about health as a fate across sovereign states. Governance, on the other hand, tries to formulate and practice stable policies and methods for public health practice within the bounds of treaty law. Because governance does not occur within the political scene, it is not subject to the divisions and deliberations of the political (Singer & Weir 2008: 57). And whereas the political scene has a specific institutional location where political divisions are articulated, governmental processes are not institutionally bound. For instance, emergency vigilance at WHO extends into global networks such as GOARN.

As the global emergency vigilance apparatus was being fashioned at the turn of the 21st century, the sovereign states that comprised WHO's members agreed to redefine their common fate with respect to the transmission of infectious diseases and the new category of international public health emergencies. The resulting legal changes in the IHR (2005) located the ultimate place of power for declaring international public health emergencies in WHO rather than sovereign states. Legally enabling WHO to gather information from unofficial sources and granting WHO the power to announce emergencies without a sovereign state's consent also disarticulated epidemiological governance knowledge from ultimate sovereign control. The politico-juridical relations of global emergency vigilance in the IHR (2005) recognize conditions where sovereign control of infectious disease information must be sacrificed for common international protection. In this sacrifice WHO acquired capacities that exceed sovereign power.

Conclusion

The rise of global emergency vigilance was from the first motivated by a political demand from the global North that was posed in terms of international EID containment. This political demand gave rise to an epistemological shift in infectious disease control, expanding its target from a small number of infectious diseases to the openness of international public health emergencies; requiring that detection of emergencies be accomplished in real time; inventing surface, event-based surveillance/monitoring techniques and aligning them with deep, case-based surveillance; and giving WHO responsibility for the public health effects of chemical, biological, radiological, and nuclear weapons use, a responsibility that had formerly been defined as a security matter outside the public health mandate of WHO. The epistemological shift resulted in the emancipation of epidemiological knowledge about public health events and international public health emergencies from ultimate sovereign control. The IHR (2005) constituted WHO as a suprasovereign power in speech acts, a power that incentivized sovereign cooperation, and gave WHO's governance apparatus expanded scope for action and innovation. After a period of pure governance in violation of a law that was treated as no longer in force by all the sovereign states that were WHO members, WHO was constituted as a global political power.

The main significance of emergency vigilance for global biopolitics has been twofold: (1) the transformation of WHO into a suprasovereign power in health; and (2) the fashioning of a governance apparatus capable of detecting and responding to international health emergencies in real time. From this analysis it may be concluded that emergency vigilance is a complex biopolitical strategy that is comprised of governance, sovereignty, and suprasovereign power. It is a form of public health knowledge articulated to but released from sovereignty, though not from the political. More generally, the case of global emergency vigilance shows the importance of investigating and reflecting on the question of the political beyond governance in scholarship related to historical and contemporary biopolitics.

6 Concluding

This book was occasioned by the 2002/2003 international SARS outbreak, particularly the actions taken by WHO in relation to Toronto, Canada. It was the first time since the 1918 influenza pandemic that a city in Canada had faced the social, political, economic, and health repercussions of an outbreak of a previously unknown, highly infectious disease that left many of those who suffered it dead. The contrast between our local, everyday experience and SARS as an event organized extralocally across differing levels of government from city to province to nation to WHO struck us forcefully. Given that WHO was not previously a highly visible social actor centrally involved in Canadian public health, we wondered by what authority it had acted. Over the course of our research we came to understand that WHO was granted the power to issue travel advisories and global alerts during an epidemic/outbreak by the World Health Assembly in May 2003 after these powers had already been applied to Beijing, Shanxi Province, and Toronto during the SARS outbreak. Our point of entry to this book thus led from the SARS outbreak in Toronto to questions of juridical right and world order.

We set out to write a book about the major transformation in international infectious disease control that had been displayed during the global SARS outbreak. As we worked with the results of our archival, documentary, and interview research, we found ourselves continually struggling to catch up with the depth of the change that has occurred in international public health reasoning and practice since the mid-1990s. It was not until the final draft of this book that we fully realized that a fundamental revision in the place of infectious disease in public health reasoning had transpired. International infectious disease control had been incorporated in global public health security and infectious diseases in international public health emergencies. Our research thus opened to an historical break in international public health apparatuses between those of the postcolonial period and global emergency vigilance. The apparatus for epidemiological communications found in the postcolonial period targeted infectious diseases on the basis of epidemiological information that was under ultimate sovereign control. The epidemiological information was systemically incomplete and out of phase with local outbreak. The second and later apparatus, global emergency vigilance, targets international public health emergencies. WHO's knowledge of international public health emergencies is based on both official epidemiological report and online detection of unofficial outbreak information, the latter combined with outbreak verification. The two apparatuses differ in their targets, temporal forms, and articulations of surface (event-based) and depth (case-based) knowledge.

The concept of global emergency vigilance owes much to the alert and risk systems theorized by Chateauraynaud and Torny (1999) as watchful apparatuses developed by nation-states from the 1960s onwards in response to political pressure to deal with health, the environment, and industry. The result was the formation of watchful apparatuses that monitor industries to identify dangers prior to their becoming calamitous. We have preferred to use the term 'vigilance apparatus' rather than 'alert and risk apparatus' given the greater economy of the term and the prior usage of 'vigilance' in public health to mean attentiveness and watchfulness. We have extended the concept of vigilance apparatus to a new empirical site, international public health, which is at a distance from the national European case studies of BSE, asbestos, and nuclear waste that Chateauraynaud and Torny undertook. Global emergency vigilance problematized ultimate sovereign power over all international epidemiological information. It required us to theorize the formation of a political level beyond the sovereign. Our concerns were thus more abstract than Chateauraynaud and Torny's and less interested in political argumentation around alerts than in the formation of a new level of political power. Chateauraynaud and Torny (1999) situated the national vigilance apparatuses they analyzed in democratic politics characterized by a public sphere of communications and nonstate organizations that debate and contest alerts. But no robust democratic public sphere exists at an international level for concerned debate about what form the suprasovereign political should take. Against the rich political culture surrounding alerts at the national level documented by Chateauraynaud and Torny, alerts in international infectious disease control are only exceptionally contested, as occurred during the SARS outbreak of 2002/2003 when Canada objected to the WHO global alert against Toronto (Whaley & Mansoor 2006: 33). In the case of international infectious disease control, political argument generally asks why WHO knowledge of and response to a potential international outbreak did not occur sooner, calling for more and better early warning detection rather than questioning early warning outbreak detection as such.

This book has offered an empirical sociology of international infectious disease control during a period when it was being reformulated as international public health security. It is a sociology fascinated by the social workings and effects of a novel public health concept—EID—the problem-space that concept introduced, and the responses to it created at the level of the technical architecture for and formal legal articulation of international public health emergencies. We have been concerned with the social organization of knowledge in global public health surveillance, in particular with the interiorization of news as a discursive resource within a new technical apparatus concerned to rapidly detect and respond to international public health emergencies. Our work here is in part an historical sociology that has engaged in comparisons of the knowledge relations formed during the period of global emergency vigilance at the turn of the 21st century with those found at WHO prior to the mid-1990s. The combined historical/sociological analytic has sharpened our understanding of the historical break in international public health reasoning and practice that took place in the late 1990s as global emergency vigilance was constituted.

The beginnings of emergency vigilance are documented in Chapter 2. EID, a disease concept formulated in the USA during the period between 1989 and 1992, differed from previous public health conceptualizations of infectious disease in presupposing a constantly changing microbial world full of potential for fashioning new diseases, rather than simply reproducing existing microbial species understood as evolving so slowly that they could be taken as constant for the purposes of public health. The radical potentiality of the microbial world was interpreted as a threat to U.S. national interests. In alliance with Canada, the USA demanded that WHO change its international infectious disease control efforts so as to contain EID through early detection and rapid response. This was a demand for the invention of a new kind of international infectious disease control. The urgency that the global North felt with respect to EID acted in tandem with its concerns about bioweapons as the size and scope of the bioweapons programme in the former Soviet Union became known, with attendant fears about the spread of its materials and expertise to those who could be hostile to Northern interests.

Our account of the EID concept locates it in geopolitical power/knowledge relations rather than reading EID as a universal human problem. This situatedness does not, however, imply that the new vigilance apparatus was good or bad, only that differing geopolitical regions of the world have had and continue to have differing interests with respect to international infectious diseases. What happened in the 1990s was that the global North began to define a position of its own strong self-interest in international communicable disease control, whereas in the second half of the 20th century it had regarded communicable diseases as mainly the problems of others (internally and externally).

The strategic plan for Emerging and other Communicable Diseases Surveillance and Control (EMC)—the WHO division established in October 1995 in response to pressure from the global North—projected a fundamentally new type of infectious disease control: a 'world on alert.' We have argued that the world on alert represented the first strategic formulation of global emergency vigilance, although it was initially directed to infectious disease outbreaks rather than international public health emergencies. The world on alert had the overarching objective "to contain communicable diseases" (WHO 1996: n.p.). In the public health sense, containment means preventing the transmission of an infectious disease from an area in which it is endemic to one in which it has been declared eradicated, although it may also mean cutting off transmission of outbreak. The EMC strategic plan goes on to elaborate a strategy for securing the international containment of communicable diseases: strengthening national surveillance and control, creating a global organizational network to monitor diseases, exchanging information faster through digital links, fashioning national and international preparedness, and forming rapid response capacity to "contain epidemics of international importance" (WHO 1996: n.p.). Response in the world on alert is held to the standard of being at the site of outbreak within 24 hours of WHO's receiving notification. The strategic plan for a world on alert is oriented to faster and more complete surveillance knowledge than had previously existed in international public health, a new institutional form of international cooperation, and rapid field response to contain outbreaks.

The world on alert is a powerful metaphor for and initial strategic sketch of global emergency vigilance. The world on alert projected a novel sociotechnical apparatus to bring outbreaks into public health knowledge and action, one that required the emancipation of public health knowledge from sovereign control and the refashioning of WHO as a suprasovereign power with a limited remit. Global emergency vigilance is an apparatus in the sense that it joins together human actors, technologies, microbial phenomena, political power, law, forms of knowledge, and organizations. Its distinctiveness lies in its epistemological, technical, and politico-juridical form.

Yet emergency vigilance might be characterized as a regime rather than an apparatus. The concept of regime has had a long association in the history of political philosophy with theorizing differing forms of organized political power. As the political philosopher Claude Lefort (1988: 2) has noted, regime in the strong sense of ancien régime "combines the idea of a type of constitution with that of a style of existence or mode of life." Bringing global emergency vigilance into the sphere of juridical right required major revisions to international public health law and posed political questions of how WHO was authorized to know about public health emergencies and where the ultimate place of power in international public health lay, whether in sovereign states or WHO. This politico-juridical change is linked to changes in daily health practices with regard to sneezing, shaking hands, constant handwashing, popular heroization of public health figures, and so forth. Emergency vigilance has become a way of life in part of the global North. Thus Global emergency vigilance could be analyzed as a regime, a project that would extend what we have investigated in the present book.

In Chapter 3 we outlined two of the most important online early warning outbreak detection systems, GPHIN and ProMED-mail, that were formed in the 1990s to provide faster and more complete international public health knowledge of outbreak and other public health events. Each uses unofficial sources of epidemiological information, bypassing sovereign control of epidemiological communications. Although public health knowledge of outbreak at WHO was comprised of official and unofficial information in the decades prior to the late 1990s, the relation between official and unofficial knowledge differs legally, politically, and socially before and after the invention of emergency vigilance. In the IHR (2005) the World Health Assembly gave WHO power to collect unofficial data about outbreak, to publicly announce an outbreak over the objections of the sovereign state in which the outbreak is occurring when information about the outbreak is already widespread, and to release global alerts and other communications. This marked an emancipation of international public health knowledge from its subordination to sovereign power.

Between 1892 and 2004 international health law targeted infectious diseases, whereas the IHR (2005) target public health emergencies of international concern. As a legal concept 'international public health emergency' includes infectious diseases but also extends to encompass foodborne illnesses and chemical, industrial, radiological, and natural disasters. International public health emergencies may be intentionally or unintentionally caused; the unintentional may be accidental or what is called 'naturally occurring.' The concept of international public health emergency conjoins previously separate areas of international law: health law concerning infectious diseases and law concerning bioweapons. Once the concept of infectious disease was displaced and encompassed by the concept of international public health emergencies, it became inaccurate to refer to the practice of containing such emergencies as infectious/communicable disease control. In the aftermath of the IHR (2005) what was formerly called communicable disease control has been increasingly termed 'public health security' or 'health security.'

The displacement of 'infectious disease' by 'international public health emergency' in international health law was accompanied by a shift in the legally authorized practices for identifying what was to be reported to WHO. From the ISR (1951) to the IHR (1969) mandatory report was required for all cases of diseases named by international treaties in infectious disease lists. The ISR (1951), for example, required sovereign states to report all cases of the following disease list: cholera, plague, relapsing fever, smallpox, typhus, and yellow fever. There is no infectious disease list in the IHR (2005), and mandatory report by the country members of WHO is therefore not organized in terms of reporting cases of a disease. Instead the IHR (2005) require report of "events which may constitute a public health emergency of international concern" that occur within their territories (IHR 2005: Art. 6). The identification of such events is stabilized through legally mandated interpretive devices intended to structure local reasoning about what to report to WHO.

The final substantive chapter of this book is a work of social and political theory that reflects on the results of our empirical work. We characterized global emergency vigilance as an epistemological shift from the period of international communicable disease control that existed at WHO from the ISR (1951) to the period between 1998 and 2000 when the first emergency vigilance apparatus was constructed. The epistemological shift has a number of characteristics. Its target, international health emergencies, is tripartite and consists of the existent, the emergent, and the potential, only some of which presently exist and can be named, unlike the infectious disease lists found in previous international health law. Emergency vigilance requires the governance of the emerging and an orientation to unknown potentialities. International public health emergencies are subject to the temporal imperative of detection in real time, whereas international public health knowledge from 1951 to the end of the 20th century was asynchronous: The story that WHO told about outbreak coincided with the local time of outbreak. The temporal standard of real-time knowledge of public health events in global emergency vigilance was made possible through the combination of unofficial and official knowledge. Unofficial knowledge is noncausal, a surface knowledge that coordinates with and incentivizes causal, depth knowledge based on case diagnoses about what is happening inside the body. In global emergency vigilance the scope of detection and response is extended well beyond infectious disease to disasters, whatever their cause, that have a public health component, that is, that involve illness or health conditions on a population/collective basis.

Global emergency vigilance was formed in the experimental space of pure governance before it was brought within the sphere of juridical right in the IHR (2005). When the global emergency vigilance apparatus was authorized by international health law, it constituted WHO as a suprasovereign power. This marked an event in global biopolitics: the constitution of a suprasovereign political level irreducible to sovereignty.

Our work on global public health emergency vigilance led us to closely consider the political in global biopolitics. There is a need for a more robust conception of biopolitics that is not reducible to governance, a practice that orients to the right disposition of people and things. Another level of the political symbolically constitutes a common fate and a common world while simultaneously instituting its continuing divisions. While Foucauldians have theorized this level of the political through an inconclusive debate about sovereign power, global emergency vigilance forces discussion of a suprasovereign political, one that is not reducible to governmentality, as sovereignty itself is not. Theorizing the political in global biopolitics requires taking into account several political forms: governance, sovereignty, and suprasovereign power. Reducing global biopolitics to governance would result in an inability to understand the significance of the distinction between the experimental, extrajudicial space in which global emergency vigilance was formed during the period between 1998 and 2003 and its inclusion within the sphere of juridical right under the IHR (2005). To conflate global biopolitics with governance would be to refuse to recognize and conceptualize some of the most difficult problems of world order in our present.

Global Public Health Vigilance creates a new analytic space for social science research on public health, particularly in the area of infectious disease and public health emergencies. We have moved in a different direction from an established analytic focus on infectious disease and public representation that has been one of the most significant forms of engagement with public health on the part of social science, cultural studies, and the humanities. One recent example of work in this tradition is Priscilla Wald's (2008) *Contagious: Cultures, Carriers, and the Outbreak Narrative,* which undertakes a narrative analysis of public discourse about 20th century infectious disease outbreaks in the USA. Outbreak narratives, Wald writes, imagine and reimagine the form of global modernity. She treats outbreak narrative as a story of heroic triumph in the face of epidemic disease, a resounding affirmation of human interdependence challenged by microbes that threaten and test that very interdependence. *Contagious* is particularly interesting in its treatment of how the press translated for popular audiences scientific concepts such as the human carrier of disease. Wald's book is part of an important analytic tradition that engages in critical reflection about the history of public discourse about epidemics. However, this tradition does little to encourage reflection on public health as an institution, about its forms of social organization, social action, knowledge relations, and practices for responding to outbreak domestically and internationally. It is unable to move past the treatment of news as representation to explore how news enters into public health practices in, for example, early warning outbreak detection.

Cultural studies approaches to public discourse on infectious disease tend also to exteriorize public health, placing its operations in a black box relevant only for its outputs with respect to public representation. We have followed a generation of science and technology studies in having an urge to open up black boxes, a practice that directs sociological attention to the workings of international public health, particularly its constitutive knowledge practices. The traditions from which we work, the history of the present and studies in the social organization of knowledge, lead to curiosity about truthful expertise and its historical effectivity, investigations into knowledge relations and ruling.

Global Public Health Vigilance has drawn Foucauldian research on public health into a dialogue with social organization of knowledge perspectives, a move that sensitizes the Foucauldian aspect of our work to knowledge relations. The theoretical idea of the active concept is a product of the dialogue between these research traditions in which we have engaged. We have decisively broken with the problematic of much Foucauldian work in public health that has privileged the neoliberal, active subject. Returning to the work of Delaporte and Foucault on the history of public health, we have sought to revitalize the sociological study of public health, to move it away from health promotion, a strategy that has been marginalized in contemporary domestic and international public health. Our work here has instead examined one of the main shifts in recent public health practice, the invention of a global public health emergency vigilance apparatus, and theorized it as a historical break from the period of international infectious disease control at WHO prior to the late 1990s.

These chapters have extended the work of a large body of scholarship from international relations, law, and political science that addresses recent changes in international infectious disease control. We have attended to the social character of the forms of knowledge that coordinate global public health practices. This aspect of our work arises from the research tradition known as studies in the social organization of knowledge. Our focus on global surveillance of public health events extends studies in the social organization of knowledge to a new empirical research site. We have analyzed a remarkable series of innovations in the concepts and reasoning that shape public health action in relation to public health emergencies. These concepts include new, emerging, and re-emerging infectious disease (EID), public health emergencies of international concern, event, and public health security. Our analysis sheds light on the textual practices through which these concepts have been mobilized and brought to bear on public health practice, drawing particular attention to the recontextualization of EID as a global concept in a sequence of reports, and the activation of public health event and public health emergencies of international concern in a new legal framework governing global emergency vigilance. Throughout, our interest has been to underscore the active character of this new conceptual landscape in the sense of its central importance for organizing a new apparatus of detection, alert, and response whose target transcends infectious disease. This emphasis has extended the existent legal studies and political science literature focused on international infectious disease control by demonstrating the relationship between developments in a formal discourse of knowledge and the possibilities and forms of international public health practice.

One of the challenges in writing a book on international public health is that it is a complex and rapidly changing field that requires constant research updates. It also requires the development of concepts and theory that are sufficiently abstract and robust that they do not require constant updating. Recently, Larry Brilliant, CEO of Google, announced his plans to produce "a GPHIN on steroids" called Innovating Support to Emergencies Diseases and Disasters (InSTEDD) and—launched its Website (http://instedd.org/). InSTEDD seeks to move beyond GPHIN to establish an independent open-source system with broader search and analysis capabilities, more languages, instant messaging and text messaging, and high-resolution coordinated satellite photography to enhance early disease detection and response (see http://www.lunchoverip.com/2006/03/can_theinterne.html). Whoever works on global public health today will be faced with the challenges of dealing with late-breaking news that may or may not be of sociological significance.

There is a clear need for more social science work about international public health. This is not just a matter of keeping abreast of a changing field but of investigating and developing more complex understandings of topics that we have not fully explored here. We close with some suggestions for such work.

This book is empirically focused on the activities of GPHIN and WHO headquarters in Geneva, with additional historical treatment of the EID concept and epidemiological communications at WHO prior to the late 1990s. But global emergency vigilance has multiple institutions, actors, and forms of expertise operating in and across many sovereign states that are differently positioned with respect to emerging imperatives to create a world on alert. Researching global health vigilance from other empirical/geographical sites would create new insights. One of these sites would be GOARN, whose work has been barely mentioned here. A line of investigation exploring the relationship between event detection and GOARN's work of mobilizing international responses to contain public health emergencies would strengthen the institutional analysis of international public health and global emergency vigilance that our focus on knowledge and knowledge relations attended to weakly. This type of investigation would need field research, which is beyond the archival, documentary, and key informant methods that we used.

Studies are needed of political responses to the role that news and the Internet now play in global public health practice. We have explored how online news has challenged sovereign control over domestic public health events and, when interiorized within the new technical apparatus of emergency vigilance, made possible rapid detection of and response to infectious disease outbreaks and other public health threats. This means that the Internet currently establishes the technical limit of the effectiveness of early warning outbreak detection. If unofficial reports are not made in electronic form, they are not searchable. One would also be naïve if one were to understand virtual global health news as a free, democratic space. As discussed in Chapter 3 there is evidence that some states—North and South—have moved to censor news coverage of local outbreaks of infectious disease, and some news reporters have been harassed for reporting stories about sensitive domestic public health events. Social scientists need to engage in ongoing efforts to understand the possibilities and limits of news and Internet sources as discursive sources of global emergency vigilance.

One of the longstanding criticisms of international infectious disease control, renewed as the emergency vigilance apparatus authorized by the IHR (2005) is being put in place, is that it is directed by the global North to its benefit. An example of this kind of critique occurs in a

recent article by Sara Davies (2008: 296) who, in the context of arguing that infectious disease has been redefined as a security matter in the
global North, notes that "[d]eveloping states have been noticeable in this
process only by their absence as key actors." Emergency vigilance, it is
said, follows a long history of colonial and neocolonial relations of international infectious disease control fuelled by anxieties about 'tropical'
diseases, with control strategies that were designed to protect Europe
and North America. After the initial funding of national core capacity
requirements in surveillance and response have been funded by public
and private donors from the global North (mandated under the IHR
[2005]), ongoing operating costs of national programmes in the global
South will need to be shouldered by countries with weak primary public
health infrastructures. A related critique is that the IHR, early warning
outbreak detection, and rapid-response tactics do very little to prevent
outbreaks in the first place through the development of better nutrition,
housing, and primary health care.

Global emergency vigilance aims to contain outbreak either by control
at national borders or, increasingly, by containment at source. It can be
argued that this is in the interest of global South nations as they can
suffer harsh economic consequences in terms of trade and international
travel. Obijiofor Aginam (2004) has also argued that the SARS outbreak
formed a model of international public health intervention that recognized the mutual vulnerability to infectious diseases of all humans in
both the South and the North, a model that goes beyond the longstanding Euro-American focus of international public health on "invasive
tropical diseases" since the mid-19th century.

The effects of global emergency vigilance on the countries of the global
South require investigation. Social science research should be undertaken
that carefully analyzes the implementation of the provisions of the revised
IHR. What have been the effects on countries of the global South? Where
have the resources come from to meet the notification and response requirements of the revised IHR? What are the effects of funding global emergency
vigilance on other national public health priorities in the countries of the
global South? In the USA, a country of the global North to be sure, many
have argued that increased funding for civilian biodefense has directed
resources into rapid-response and public health preparedness and away
from routine public health activities and longer-term approaches to public
health problems (Packard, Brown, Berkelman, & Frumkin 2004; Stoto,
Schonlau, & Mariano 2004).

The relations between public health and security are complex, if only
because security has so many meanings and practices. On the one hand,
public health security may be used in the sense of reducing acute threats
to health among vulnerable populations (WHO 2007: 3). On the other
hand, public health at national and international levels is being integrated with biosecurity, the protection of national populations and the

international system against threats from infectious diseases and bioweapons (Davies 2008; Fidler & Gostin 2008; McInnes & Lee 2006). Our own work here has mainly considered emergency vigilance in relation to biosecurity, beginning in the discussion of the invention of the EID concept and its articulation to U.S. national security interests. In Chapter 3, we showed that the detection of bioweapons use has been integrated into the design of the online early warning outbreak detection systems GPHIN and ProMED-mail. Chapter 5 demonstrated that the very definition of "disease" in the IHR (2005) was adapted for application to the deliberate and accidental spread of chemical, biological, and radiological weapons: "'Disease' means an illness or medical condition, irrespective of origin or sources, that present or could present significant harm to humans" (IHR 2005: Art. 1). In previous international health law, infectious disease was presumed to be an event independent of human will. In the IHR (2005), international public health emergencies are proximate to human agency, whether accidentally caused, deliberate, or the unintended result of human practices in relation to environment and animals. The legal concept of 'international public health emergencies' was designed to enable WHO-organized interventions in the public health aspects of bioweaspons use, but also chemical and radiological agents, unlike all previous international health law (Fidler & Gostin 2008: 138).

The effects of securitizing on local, national and global public health need investigation. The effects of international and national emergency vigilance regimes on communicable disease prevention and control require careful documentation. The impact of funding civilian biodefense programmes on public health systems may pose some of the same problems for public health systems of the global North that vertical, disease-specific development assistance for health has had for the countries of the global South when public health workers are drawn into better paying jobs. Generally speaking, the integration of some aspects of public health into emergency planning needs scholars to ask questions. The research terrain is open.

In this book we have entered two social science schools into dialogue—the history of the present into dialogue with studies in the social organization of knowledge—to explore the historical formation and organization of a new global public health emergency vigilance apparatus. That apparatus represents the refashioning of international infectious disease control, as a practice of public health security, a revision of its primary target of intervention from infectious desease to international public health emergencies, a transformation of public health surveillance throughout the emergence of unofficial information as functionally parallel to official epidemiological report, and the emergence of WHO as a suprasovereign power. We hope that the analytic and research directions we have established in this book elicit more work in the area. There is much more to be known about emergency vigilance, much more to contribute to a revitalized sociology of public health.

Notes

NOTES TO CHAPTER 1

· 1. 'Infectious disease' and 'communicable disease' will be treated as synonymous here, as they are in Last's *A Dictionary of Epidemiology* (Last 2001). Each term has been in use throughout the 20th century. The Medline Plus Medical Dictionary makes a slight difference between infectious disease as a disease caused by invasive microbes versus communicable disease as a subset of infectious diseases distinguished by its form of transmission: "Infectious disease: a disease caused by the entrance into the body of organisms (as bacteria, protozoans, fungi, or viruses) which grow and multiply there"; "Communicable disease: an infectious disease transmissible (as from person to person) by direct contact with an affected individual or the individual's discharges or by indirect means (as by a vector)." Retrieved February 6, 2009, from http://www.nlm.nih.gov/medlineplus/mplusdictionary.html. http://www2.merriam-webster.com/cgi-bin/mwmednlm?book=Medical&va=

2. For example, see the definition of public health surveillance in the report of the CDC Guidelines Working Group, *Updated Guidelines for Evaluating Public Health Surveillance Systems*: "Public health surveillance is the ongoing systematic collection, analysis, interpretation, and dissemination of data regarding a health-related event for use in public health action to reduce morbidity and mortality to improve health" (CDC Guidelines Working Group 2001: 2).

3. We thank our colleague Fuyuki Kurasawa (Department of Sociology, York University, Toronto) for sharing with us his recent work in association with Daniel Cefaï (Department of Sociology, University of Paris 10) on what they have called "pragmatic" sociology in contemporary France.

NOTES TO CHAPTER 2

1. The internal text citation "Lac Tremblant Declaration" is to "Proceedings and Recommendations of the Expert Working Group on Emerging Infectious Disease Issues: Lac Tremblant Declaration."

2. See the Nobel Prize biography of Lederberg. Retrieved November 26, 2007, from http://nobelprize.org/nobel_prizes/medicine/laureates/1958/lederberg-bio.html. For an overview of Lederberg's work on EID from the perspective of the CDC, see Hughes & Drotman (2008).

3. Compare, for instance, the words of Dr. Alexander Primrose in his Chair's address to the Canadian Medical Association in 1925 on the double-edged nature of "modern means of transportation":

It is impossible to overestimate the revolutionary effect of modern methods of transportation on our national life. Quick transportation by sea
and land, more recently in the air, with added comfort in travel, has
induced an ever increasing number of people to go abroad. A continuous
stream of travelers passes from one country to another. Not only so, but
there is a constant interchange of commodities including food stuffs and
the transportation of cattle. The most important factor to be considered,
however, is the movement of immigrants. It is no longer possible for any
nation to remain isolated and self-contained: the destiny of each country
is inevitably affected by its relations to other countries. This fact was
demonstrated and forced upon the attention of the national of the world
during the great war and its aftermath. (Primrose 1925: 246)

In the last sentence of this citation Primrose was clearly alluding to the
1918 influenza epidemic as an instance of global interconnectedness.

4. WHO's shoestring budget is mentioned several times in *Emerging Viruses*
   (Morse 1993) and *Emerging Infections* (IOM 1992). Contributors to the
   Morse collection quote a WHO official as having said that the annual budget of WHO was less than that of a U.S. general hospital (Letgers, Brink, &
   Takafuji 1993: 276), which made it difficult for WHO to fund new programming for international response to infectious diseases. Nowhere in either
   volume was any acknowledgement made that the USA was in arrears on its
   payments to WHO. On the history of U.S. debt to the U.N. system to 1996,
   see UNA-USA (1997).
5. "Stephen S. Morse, Faculty Profile, Mailman School of Public Health."
   Retrieved June 21, 2009, from http://www.mailmanschool.org/msphfacdir/
   profile/asp?uni=ssm20.
6. See Agamben's discussion (1998: 44–48) of the theory of *dynamis/energeia*
   in Aristotle's *Metaphysics*.
7. The source material does read "complimentary," not "complementary."
8. See cover page, "Emerging and Other Communicable Diseases. Strategic Plan
   1996–2000," World Health Organization, EMC, WHO/EMC/96.1. Retrieved
   February, 2009, from whqlibdoc.who.int/hq/1997/WHO_EMC_97.3.pdf.
9. We have concentrated on the reception of the EID concept at WHO, but
   international public health of course includes many more organizations. Pan
   American Health Organization (PAHO) also received the EID concept in the
   mid-1990s, with the first PAHO conference on EID taking place in 1995. See
   Epstein 1995.
10. 49th World Health Assembly. (1996, May 20–25, Geneva, Switzerland).
    Provisional agenda item 19.2, A49/6, Add. 1 (1996, May 16), *New, emerg-*
    ing, and re-emerging infectious diseases, and revision of the International
    Health Regulations: 2. Unpublished document, WHO Library: Geneva,
    Switzerland.
11. The WHO programme, Emergency Aid in Epidemics, was established in 1969
    to obtain rapid knowledge of outbreak and to control its spread ("Notes of
    a Meeting Held in Director CD's Office on 27 September 1971 Concerning
    the WHO Programme for Emergency Aid in Epidemics." WHO Archives,
    WHO 10, Records of the Central Registry, WHO Headquarters: Sub-fonds 3
    1955–1983, Emergency Aid in Epidemics, C8/180/2). During the 1970s there
    was a conceptual tension between "emergency aid in epidemics" and other
    aspects of WHO programming, in particular multiyear planning and disease
    prevention. The Fifth General Programme of Work (for the period from 1973
    to 1977) made clear that emergencies were exceptions to what it considered
    to be rational public health planning. The usual course of events should be
    "the investigation of the natural histories of communicable diseases with

a view to their more rationally planned control" (WHO 1971: 67). Thus emergency aid was held to be sometimes at odds with investment in communicable disease prevention. What constituted aid was also interpreted as sometimes extending into what usually would be termed prevention. In 1969, during consultations prior to the formation of Emergency Aid in Epidemics, the Chief of Environmental Health at WHO noted that a specialist in environmental health might arguably have several tasks in an epidemic, including "to study, develop and implement a broader and more long-term programme which will help in curtailing similar epidemics; or for alleviating the conditions brought about by a disaster" (Memorandum from Chief, Environmental Health, to Dr. N.F. Izmerov, ADG. [1969, July 25]. Subject: "Emergency Aid in Epidemics." WHO Archives, WHO 10, Records of the Central Registry, WHO Headquarters: Sub-fonds 3 1955–1983, Emergency Aid in Epidemics, C8/180/2.)

12. On the ethical complexities of the duty to treat under conditions of epidemic infectious disease, see the August 2008 issue of *The American Journal of Bioethics*.

13. In November 2007, the Division of Communicable Diseases (the successor to EMC) was reorganized and renamed Health Security and Environment. This change was motivated by the expanded responsibilities of WHO in relation to public health emergencies of international concern. Health Security and Environment "includes the department of Epidemic and Pandemic Alert and Response (EPR) with the addition of the Cholera team and the team on Disease Control in Humanitarian Emergencies, the department of Protection of the Human Environment (PHE) and the department of Food Safety, Zoonoses and Foodborne Diseases (FOS). The changes within this cluster reflect the expanded scope of the International Health Regulations (2005), which include emergencies caused by chemicals and other environmental hazards and outbreaks of foodborne disease . . ." (IHR News 2007).

14. 'Holoendemic' disease is an epidemiological term for infection that begins for the most part during childhood and that most children in a given population have. A disease that is termed holoendemic has greater prevalence in children than adults.

15. PEPFAR has been widely criticized for making its funding contingent upon commitments on the part of recipients to abstinence-based HIV/AIDS prevention, restricted distribution of condoms, and explicit disavowal of sex work. See, for example, Health Gap (2006); "PEPFAR and the Fight against AIDS" (2007).

16. World Bank MAP, Multi-Country HIV/AIDS Program. Retrieved July 3, 2009, from http://web.worldbank.org/WBSITE/EXTERNAL/COUN-TRIES/AFRICAEXT/EXTAFRHEANUTPOP/EXTAFRREGTOPHIVAI DS/0,,contentMDK:20415735~menuPK:1001234~pagePK:34004173~piP K:34003707~theSitePK:717148,00.html#GOALS.

17. For governments and agencies included in this estimate, see OECD-DAC (2008: Table 1A).

18. MacKellar (2005: 309) concludes an important empirical study of the extent to which official development assistance has or has not matched the stated health priorities of recipient countries by noting "the absence of a clear relationship between how health is treated in the preparation of poverty-reduction strategies and the composition of development assistance."

19. See the key planning document "Scaling up for Better Health: Work Plan for the International Health Partnership and Related Initiatives (IHP+)." Retrieved November 5, 2008, from http://www.internationalhealthpartner-ship.net/pdf/02_IHP_Workplan_EN_Feb20_2008_FINAL.pdf.

20. The relevant sessions included the following: "HIV and Human Resources: Competing Priorities or Interconnected Solutions," noncommercial satellite session, August 3, XVIII International AIDS Conference 2008; "Global Financial Architecture," special session (TUSS01), August 5, XVIII International AIDS Conference 2008; "Positive Synergies Between Health Systems and Global Health Initiatives," noncommercial satellite session (MOSAT16), August 4, XVIII International AIDS Conference 2008; "Global Health Initiatives: The Impact of Vertical Funding on Health Systems and Community Priorities," oral abstract session (TUAX02) August 5, XVIII International AIDS Conference 2008; "HIV/AIDS Donor Interactions with the National Health System in Mozambique, Uganda and Zambia," noncommercial satellite session (WESAT12), August 6, XVIII International AIDS Conference 2008; and "Strengthening the Health System through the AIDS Response," special session, (THSS02), August 7, XVIII International AIDS Conference 2008.

NOTES TO CHAPTER 3

1. The Far Eastern Bureau broadcasts included not only case and mortality data on the quarantinable diseases (plague, cholera, and smallpox) that were mandated under international public health law, but also a variety of information related to other diseases thought due to infection, along with quarantine regulations and equipment in ports, the health of pilgrims, and STDs in seafarers (Manderson 1995: 123). The Far Eastern Bureau telegraphic code included a section on "Infectious Disease" that was divided into two subsections, the first on "disease nomenclature and prevalence" that contained a list of 46 diseases and the second subsection on "general epidemiological intelligence" (Brooke 1926).
2. Alison Bashford (2004: 134–135) has documented the reception in Australia of the Far Eastern Bureau's weekly reports.
3. The transference from colonial to national control of epidemiological intelligence was within the memory of a respondent to one of Dr. Karel Raška's papers on the surveillance of communicable diseases. (Dr. Raška was Director of the Division of Communicable Diseases at WHO headquarters during the 1960s.) The respondent, B. Traore, noted that in West Africa "[a]t the time of independence, there was in each country a coordinated system and this Service covered French West Africa and even Togo. But with independence, there began a process of 'balkanization'—each country went into its ivory tower to taste the fruit of independence" (Raška 1968: Discussion, 413). After the incidence of certain infectious diseases rose in West Africa, a regional organization was formed: Society for a Joint Campaign against the Major Endemic Diseases (Raška 1968: Discussion, 413). B. Traore's remarks traced an historical trajectory that led from a colonial epidemiological intelligence system to national systems, followed by international cooperation at a regional level.
4. The Interim Commission of the World Health Organization was a transitional body administering initial WHO operations and the last work of the League of Nations Health Organisation between the formal establishment of WHO in 1946 and the ratification of the WHO Constitution on April 7, 1948.
5. WHO Archives, WHO 10, Records of the Central Registry, WHO Headquarters, Sub-fonds 1, Information on Use of Current Methods of Epidemiological Reporting, Microfilm: 452-1-3.
6. Ibid., Part I, Question III, "Table of Suggestions for the Creation of a Unified Epidemiological Information Service": 26–27.

7. Memorandum of Dr. L. Bernard, ADG, to Director-General Candau (1971, December 15). Subject: "Discontinuation of the Daily Epidemiological Radiotelegraphic Bulletin." WHO Archives, WHO 10, Records of the Central Registry, WHO Headquarters: Sub-fonds 3 1955–1984: Epidemiological Radio Bulletins: General Information, E7/415/1.

8. Memorandum of Dr. Ian D. Carter, ESCD, to Dr. E. Roelsgaard, Chief ESCD (1971, December 8). Subject: "Daily Epidemiological Radiotelegraphic Bulletin." WHO Archives, WHO 10, Records of the Central Registry, WHO Headquarters: Sub-fonds 3 1955–1984: Epidemiological Radio Bulletins: General Information, E7/415/1.

9. Ibid.

10. "The Maldives' Ordeal by Cholera." (1978, May 3). *The Statesman*, WHO Archives, WHO 10, Records of the Central Registry, WHO Headquarters: Sub-fonds 3 1955–1983: Emergency Situations—Cholera Outbreak—S.E. Asian Region, C6/180/2.

11. Telegram from Malafatapoulos "urgent director/cos." (1978, April 25). WHO Archives, WHO 10, Records of the Central Registry, WHO Headquarters: Sub-fonds 3 1955–1983: Emergency Situations—Cholera Outbreak—S.E. Asian Region, C6/180/2.

12. Memorandum of Dr. P. Brès, Chief, VIR, to Dr. I.D. Ladnyi, ADG. (1977, December 20). Subject: "Rift Valley Fever Outbreak in Egypt." WHO Archives, WHO 10, Records of the Central Registry, WHO Headquarters: Sub-fonds 3 1955–1983: WHO Emergency Aid in Epidemics, C8/180/2.

13. Ibid.

14. Telex of Dr. A. Pio, CDS Unisanté Geneva to Unisanté Alexandria. (1987, March 17). WHO Archives, WHO 10, Records of the Central Registry, WHO Headquarters: Sub-fonds 3 1955–1983: WHO Emergency Aid in Epidemics, C8/180/2. The text we quote and attribute to W.R. Jakarta is prefaced in Dr. Pio's telex with the words "Following information from W.R. Jakarta quote."

15. The unpublished field investigation report was titled "Children's Mortality in Naples: Progress Report." (1979, February 12, Rome). WHO Archives, WHO 10, Records of the Central Registry, WHO Headquarters: Sub-fonds 3 1955–1983: WHO Emergency Aid in Epidemics, C8/180/2.

16. Letter from Dr. Ian Carter, Medical Officer in Epidemiological Surveillance of Communicable Diseases, to Dr. L. Pudegia (spelling of proper name unclear in document), Chief Officer, Laboratory Services, Bir Hospital, Kathmandu (Nepal), (1977, August 24). WHO Archives, WHO 10, Records of the Central Registry, WHO Headquarters: Sub-fonds 3 1955–1983, Outbreaks of Diarrhoeal Diseases Including Cholera—South-East Asian Region, C6/180/2SE.

17. "Prétendue Flambée Épidemique en Algérie," AFRO-WHOGRAM—PRIORITY, to WR, Algérie, from Dr. E.G. Beausoleil, Chef de Programme, Lutte contre la Maladie pour le Directeur regional. (1987, January 29). WHO Archives, WHO 10, Records of the Central Registry, WHO Headquarters: Sub-fonds 3 1955–1983, Outbreaks of Diarrhoeal Diseases including Cholera—African Region, C6/180/2AF.

18. Telegram from H. Mahler, M.D., Director-General, to Health Minister, Addis Ababa. (1985, April 22). WHO Archives, WHO 10, Records of the Central Registry, WHO Headquarters: Sub-fonds 3 1955–1983, Outbreaks of Diarrhoeal Diseases including Cholera—African Region, C6/180/2AF. After the first two sentences reproduced here, the telegram states:
    Believe that this situation is a good example of how you can make maximum use of your WHO in order to ensure the health of the people of Ethiopia

and to limit trade and economic restrictions. Accordingly would humbly suggest that a WHO expert visit Ethiopia to collaborate with you in assessing epidemiological situation and in determining related supply needs which I believe can be mobilized. Such collaboration would be consistent with that being provided during the past few years by WHO to your national diarrhoeal disease control programme. Grateful your reply by cable or telephone soonest. Mahler Unisanté Geneva.

19. "Telex to all Regional Directors" from Epidnations. (n.d.). WHO Archives, WHO 10, Records of the Central Registry, WHO Headquarters: Sub-fonds 3 1955–1983, Outbreaks of Diarrhoeal Diseases Including Cholera—African Region, C6/180/2AF. The date this telex was sent is likely late August 1970 as it appears amidst documents of this date dealing with the cholera outbreak in the Middle East and Africa.

20. Telex from Dr. P. Dorolle to Director-General Candau. (1970, August 28). WHO Archives, WHO 10, Records of the Central Registry, WHO Headquarters: Sub-fonds 3, 1955–1983: Outbreaks of Diarrhoeal Diseases Including Cholera—African Region, C6/180/2AF.

21. Telex from Dr. P. Dorolle to Director-General Candau. (1970, August 28). WHO Archives, WHO 10, Records of the Central Registry, WHO Headquarters: Sub-fonds 3, 1955–1983, Outbreaks of Diarrhoeal Diseases Including Cholera—African Region, C6/180/2AF.

22. Letter from Dr. Pierre Dorolle, ADG, to Ambassador J. Fernand-Laurent, Permanent Representative of France at the WHO. (1979, September 1). WHO Archives, WHO 10, Records of the Central Registry, WHO Headquarters: Sub-fonds 3 1955–1983: Outbreaks of Diarrhoeal Diseases Including Cholera—African Region, C6/180/2AF. Ambassador Fernand-Laurent's letter is quoted in Dr. Dorolle's response.

23. Letter of Dr. P. Dorolle, WHO Deputy Director-General, to United States Mission to the United National Office and other International Organizations at Geneva. (1970, August 31). WHO Archives, WHO 10, Records of the Central Registry, WHO Headquarters: Sub-fonds 3 1955–1983, Outbreaks of Diarrhoeal Diseases Including Cholera—African Region, C6/180/2AF. Dr. Dorolle's letter responded to a letter from the United States Mission signed by Jesse L. Steinfeld, Surgeon of the Public Health Service of the United States of America, dated August 31, 1970. The passage reproduced here is an extract from Steinfeld's letter quoted by Dorolle.

24. Letter of Dr. P. Dorolle, WHO Deputy Director-General, to United States Mission to the United National Office and other International Organizations at Geneva. (1970, August 31). WHO Archives, WHO 10, Records of the Central Registry, WHO Headquarters: Sub-fonds 3 1955–1983, Outbreaks of Diarrhoeal Diseases Including Cholera—African Region, C6/180/2AF. Dr. Dorolle's letter quotes the response of the Director-General to the letter from the United States Mission signed by Dr. Steinfeld. (See Note 22).

25. "Cholera and Politics." (1970, September 3). *The New York Times*, WHO Archives, WHO 10, Records of the Central Registry, WHO Headquarters: Sub-fonds 3, 1955–1983, Outbreaks of Diarrhoeal Diseases Including Cholera—African Region, C6/180/2AF.

26. WHO, "Strategies for the Control of Emergencies Caused by Epidemics of Communicable Diseases" (informal consultation, November 9–13, 1981: Geneva, Switzerland). Section F: Information: An Active Role in Emergencies: 1. CDS/Mtg./WP/81.18. Unpublished document, WHO Library: Geneva, Switzerland.

27. Ibid.

28. Ibid.

29. WHO, "Strategies for the Control of Emergencies Caused by Epidemics of Communicable Diseases" (informal consultation, November 9–13, 1981: Geneva, Switzerland). WHO Global Emergency Services: 2. CDS/ Mtg./WP/81.15: p. 2. Unpublished document, WHO Library: Geneva, Switzerland.

30. Ibid. and WHO, "Strategies for the Control of Emergencies Caused by Epidemics of Communicable Diseases" (informal consultation, November 9–13, 1981: Geneva, Switzerland). Section F: Information: An Active Role in Emergencies: p. 1. CDS/Mtg./WP/81.18. Unpublished document, WHO Library: Geneva, Switzerland.

31. Passive surveillance systems are based on case reports mandated by law and received from physicians and other personnel in accordance with the terms of the law. In active surveillance, data collection is done by contacting physicians and other relevant parties to obtain case and event data (Brookmeyer & Stroup 2004: 168).

32. Indians panic over plague—200,000 flee city where disease has killed at least 24. (1994, Sept. 24) *Sun Sentinel*, p. 17A.

33. GPHIN uses revenue from subscriptions exclusively to fund the development and enhancement of the GPHIN system (GPHIN Interview).

34. GPHIN member, personal communication, January 27, 2009.

35. The Federation of American Scientists is a center of policy research and analysis focused on science and technology dimensions of global issues. The organization was founded by scientists who worked on the Manhattan Project to develop the first atomic bomb. It has a strong focus on disarmament and is currently sponsored by some 70 Nobel Laureates (Madoff & Woodall 2005; Federation of American Scientists, "About FAS," retrieved on December 10, 2008, from http://www.fas.org/about/index.html).

36. "About ProMED-mail." Retrieved on December 23, 2008, from http://www.promedmail.org/pls/otn/f?p=2400:1950:6331310215202::NO:::.

37. ProMED-mail has a main list as well as specific e-mail distribution lists for particular geographic regions (e.g., Portuguese and Spanish lists for Latin America) and for specific topic areas such as animal diseases and plant diseases (Madoff 2005).

38. With the intention to stabilize funding, GPHIN is currently considering moving to a user access system that would reduce or eliminate paid subscriptions.

39. See the HealthMap Web site for information about its funding. Retrieved June 15, 2009, from http://www.healthmap.org.

40. Predicting and tracking pandemics: HealthMap.org tracking H1N1 flu hot spots in real time. (2009, April 30). *Medicine & Health/Diseases*. Retrieved June 15, 2009, from http://www.physorg.com/news160325542.html.

41. See the entry "monitoring" in Last's *A Dictionary of Epidemiology* (Last 2001):
    The intermittent performance and analysis of routine measurements, aimed at detecting changes in the environment or health status of populations. Not to be confused with surveillance which is a continuous process. To some, monitoring also implies intervention in the light of observed measurements.

42. WHO "Coordinated rapid outbreak response." Retrieved December 20, 2008, from http://www.who.int/csr/alertresponse/rapidresponse/en/index.html.

43. Global health security: epidemic alert and response (World Health Assembly document A54/9). (2001). Geneva, Switzerland: World Health Organization.

44. The *Weekly Epidemiological Record* is available online at http://www.who. int/wer/en/
45. The longer quotation from the GPHIN research participant may be of interest. S/he used the powerful metaphor of pyramid and flat plane to conceptualize the effects of outbreak detection on official information: "We were squashing the pyramid down to flat plane in which information could come from any particular place at any time. And governments were no longer in control of their information." "Pyramid" refers to the "pyramid of report" in official epidemiological reporting wherein case information flows from local to regional to national to international public health authorities. This research participant contrasts the pyramid of official report to the "flat plane" of GPHIN that sources information beyond sovereign control.
46. "The 1998 ProMED-mail Award for Excellence in Outbreak Reporting on the Internet." Retrieved September 28, 2008, from http://www.promedmail. org/pls/otn/wwv_flow.accept.

NOTES TO CHAPTER 4

1. 'States Parties' is the legal term used to refer to WHO country members under the IHR. All WHO States Parties are subject to the terms of the IHR (2005) unless they opt out. None had done so by December 15, 2006, the deadline for opting out. Only a few States Parties have formally expressed reservations (WHO 2008b).
2. International Sanitary Convention, January 30, 1892, 176 Cons. T.S., 395 at 399. The 1892 International Sanitary Convention more presupposes than explicitly defines that it is an agreement about dealing only with cholera. The ratifications section of this Convention anticipated extending international agreements to cover plague and yellow fever, delegating the responsibility for the revisions to the Conseil Sanitaire, Maritime, et Quarantenaire d'Égypte (ibid.: 398).
3. International Sanitary Convention, March 19, 1897, 184 Cons. T.S. 264 at 274.
4. International Sanitary Convention, January 17, 1912, 215 Cons. T.S. 223 at 228.
5. "Notes of a Meeting Held in Director CD's Office on 27 September 1971 Concerning the WHO Programme for Emergency Aid in Epidemics." WHO Archives, WHO 10, Records of the Central Registry, WHO Headquarters: Sub-fonds 3 1955–1984: Emergency Aid in Epidemics, C8/180/2.
6. Memorandum of Chief, VIR, to Director, CD. (1971, October 20). Subject: "WHO Scheme for Emergency Aid in Epidemics." WHO Archives, WHO 10, Records of the Central Registry, WHO Headquarters: Sub-fonds 3 1955–1984: Emergency Aid in Epidemics, C8/180/C2, p. 3. The annual expenditures for Emergency Aid in Epidemics during 1970 were US$374,083 and US$12,508 in 1971 (to Oct. 21). See Memorandum of Director CD to Dr. L. Bernard, ADG. (1971, November 2). Subject: "WHO Emergency Aid in Epidemics." WHO Archives, WHO 10, Records of the Central Registry, WHO Headquarters: Sub-fonds 3 1955–1984: Emergency Aid in Epidemics, C8/180/2, p. 2.
7. Memorandum of Dr. W. Chas. Cockburn, Chief, VIR, to Dr. Payne, ADG. (1968, March 4). Subject: "Emergency Aid for Epidemics of Virus Diseases." WHO Archives, WHO 10, Records of the Central Registry, WHO Headquarters: Sub-fonds 3 1955–1984, Emergency Aid in Epidemics, C8/180/2. Cockburn's memorandum historically coincided with the occurrence of major

polio vaccination campaigns in global North. The Pan American Health Organization did leading work in polio vaccinations in the Americas.

8. Memorandum of Director CD to Dr. L. Bernard, ADG. (1971, November 2). WHO Archives, WHO 10, Records of the Central Registry, WHO Headquarters: Sub-fonds 3 1955–1984: Emergency Aid in Epidemics, C8/180/2.

9. AFRO-Memorandum of Dr. S. Malafatopoulos, Director of Health Services for the Regional Director, to Dr. K. Raška, Director CD/HQ. (1969, Feb. 14). Subject: "Consultants for Plague in Congo." WHO Archives, WHO 10, Records of the Central Registry, WHO Headquarters: Sub-fonds 3 1955–1984: Information on Plague Situation and Outbreak—Republic of Zaire, P 6/180/3. Dr. Malafatopoulos was replying to a letter from Dr. Raška stating that sending a team of two consultants to do a field investigation was "premature" given the impending rainy season and lack of laboratory support in the Democratic Republic of the Congo. Raška thought one consultant sufficient. See Dr. K. Raška, Director of CD/HQ, to Dr. A.A. Quenum, AFRO-RD. (1969, January 31). WHO Archives, WHO 10, Records of the Central Registry, WHO Headquarters: Sub-fonds 3 1955–1984: Information on Plague Situation and Outbreak—Republic of Zaire, P6/180/3.

We note that the Democratic Republic of the Congo had been left with a critical shortage of health care personnel when, in the wake of that country's independence, foreign/colonial doctors departed. WHO responded in the early 1960s with an emergency programme for training medical doctors (WHO 1968: 89–90).

10. World Health Organization. "Strategies for the Control of Emergencies Caused by Epidemics of Communicable Diseases" (informal consultation, November 9–11, 1981: Geneva, Switzerland). CDS.Mtg./82.1, p. 4. Unpublished document, WHO Library: Geneva, Switzerland.

11. Report by the Secretariat, "Revision of the International Health Regulations," WHO Executive Board, 111th Session. (2002, December 15). Provisional agenda item 5.12, EB111/34, p. 1. Unpublished document, WHO Library: Geneva, Switzerland.

12. Ibid.

13. Ibid.

14. The IHR (2005) also build in an expectation that WHO country members will communicate their experiences and difficulties with the new reporting obligations through the establishment of a new Review Committee. Reporting to the Director-General, the Review Committee has amongst its responsibilities making recommendations regarding amendments to the IHR and providing technical advice regarding their functioning.

NOTES TO CHAPTER 5

1. We would like to thank Brian Singer for his comment on the emancipation of knowledge, which we have run with here.

2. Since early warning outbreak detection also includes whatever may give rise to outbreaks of existing, emerging, and potential diseases or conditions, it may be said to have a six-part object, with three categories on two levels. We have spared readers an analysis of all six cells as the tripartite schema found here can easily be extended to the level of the conditions that might give rise to the actual, the emerging, and the potential.

3. Of course, case report data sometimes appears in the sources used by early warning outbreak detection—for instance, in news reports of hospital press

releases—but such inclusion does not overturn the general principle that the case report is not the unit of outbreak detection .

4. We will confess that there is a particularly good overview article on real-time computing in Wikipedia. "Real-time computing." Retrieved January 7, 2009, from http://en.wikipedia.org.wiki/Real-time-computing.

5. Many thanks to Fabian Voegeli for calling our attention to the significance of duration in relation to real time in its communications sense.

6. World Health Organization (WHO). WHO headquarters structure (excluding partnerships secretariats). October 22, 2008. Retrieved January 30, 2009 from www.who.int/about/hq_structure_22oct08.pdf.

7. This phrase was suggested by Brian Singer.

8. For a Foucauldian critique of Hardt and Negri's conception of biopolitics, see Rabinow and Rose (2003).

9. Dodgson et al. (2002: 6) broadly define "governance" as "the actions and means adopted by a society to promote collective action and deliver collective solutions in pursuit of common goals."

10. The expansive Foucauldian concept of 'government' differs from the 'governance' concept employed in the global health literature, however, in being restricted to the practices of expertise that seek to manage conduct, that is the savoirs normed by the distinction between the true and the false discussed in chapter 1. In contrast, global health 'governance' as it is used by Dodgson et al. (2002) is not necessarily the work of expertise.

11. Rose (1999: 15–20) provides a Foucauldian justification for preferring 'government' to sociologies of 'governance' on grounds that the study of government is concerned with "the conditions of possibility and intelligibility for certain ways of seeking to act on the conduct of others, or oneself, to achieve certain ends" (Rose 1999: 19). 'Government' is linked to a series of distinctive critical questions about expertise and truth such as what categories of person have historically has produced truth and to what ends. As the readers of our work will in part be public health personnel and health policy researchers, we have chosen to speak of 'governance' rather than 'government' because 'government' strongly indicates sovereign polities to these groups, and it has been possible to address critical questions in the context of using 'governance.'

Bibliography

Abdullah, A. S. (2007). International Health Regulations (2005). *Regional Health Forum, 11*(1), 10–16. Http://www.searo.who.int/LinkFiles/Regional_Health_Forum_IHR-2005.pdf, (retrieved 2009, October 18).

Agamben, G. (1998). *Homo sacer: Sovereign power and bare life.* Palo Alto, CA: Stanford University Press.

Agamben, G. (2005). *State of exception* (K. Attell, Trans.). Chicago and London: University of Chicago Press.

Aginam, O. (2002). International law and communicable diseases. *Bulletin of the World Health Organization, 80*(12): 946–951.

Aginam, O. (2004). Between isolationism and mutual vulnerability: A South–North perspective on global governance of epidemics in an age of globalization. *Temple Law Review, 77*(3): 296–312.

Aginam, O. (2005a). Bio-terrorism, human security and public health: Can international law bring them together in an age of globalization? *Medicine and Law, 24*: 455–62.

Aginam, O. (2005b). *Global health governance: International law and public health in a divided world.* Toronto: University of Toronto Press.

Amrith, S. S. (2006). *Decolonizing international health: India and Southeast Asia, 1930–65.* Cambridge, UK: Cambridge University Press.

Amsterdamska, O. (2005). Demarcating epidemiology. *Science, Technology & Human Values, 30*(1): 17–51.

Anghie, A. (2007). *Imperialism, sovereignty, and the making of international law.* Cambridge, UK: Cambridge University Press.

Angus, N., Jones, J., Aavitsland, P., & Giesecke, J. (2005). Proposed new International Health Regulations. *British Medical Journal, 330*: 321–322.

Armstrong D. (1983). *Political anatomy of the body: Medical knowledge in Britain in the twentieth century.* Cambridge, UK and New York: Cambridge University Press.

Armstrong, D. (1995). The rise of surveillance medicine. *Sociology of Health and Illness, 17*: 393–410.

Ashraf, H. (1999). International Health Regulations: Putting public health on the centre stage. *Lancet, 354*(9195): 2062.

Atlas, R. M., & Reppy, J. (2005). Globalizing biosecurity. *Biosecurity and Bioterrorism: Biodefense Strategy, Practice, and Science, 2*(1): 51–60.

Bal, M. (1985). *Narratology: Introduction to the theory of narrative.* Toronto, Canada: University of Toronto Press.

Barss, P. (1992). Epidemiologic field investigation as applied to allegations of chemical, biological, or toxin warfare. *Politics and the Life Sciences 11*(1): 5–22.

Barratt, A., Trevena, L., Davey, H., & McCaffery, K. (2004). Use of decision aids to support informed choices about screening. *British Medical Journal, (329)*: 507–510.

Bartelson, J. (1995). *A genealogy of sovereignty*. Cambridge, UK: Cambridge University Press.

Bashford, A. (2004). *Imperial hygiene: A critical history of colonialism, nationalism and public health*. Houndmills, Basingbroke, Hampshire, and New York: Palgrave Macmillan.

Bashford, A. (2006). Global biopolitics and the history of world health. *History of the Human Sciences*, 18(1): 67–88.

Benoist, A. D. (2008). Global terrorism and the state of permanent exception: The significance of Carl Schmitt's thought today. In L. Odysseos & F. Petito (Eds.), *The international political thought of Carl Schmitt: A new global nomos?* (pp. 73–96). London and New York: Routledge.

Berg, M. (1995). Turning a practice into a science: Reconceptualizing postwar medical practice. *Social Studies of Science*, 25: 437–476.

Berkelman, R., & Freeman, P. (2004). Emerging illness and the CDC response. In R. Packard, P. J. Brown, R. Berkelman, & H. Frumkin (Eds.), *Emerging Illnesses and Society* (pp. 350–387). Baltimore and London: Johns Hopkins University Press.

Bhattacharya, S. (2006). *Expunging variola: The control and eradication of smallpox in India, 1947–1977*. Chennai, India: Orient Longman.

Bock, G., & Thane, P. (Eds.). (1991). *Maternity and gender policies: Women and the rise of European welfare states 1880s–1950s*. London and New York: Routledge.

Brookmeyer, R., & Stroup, D.F. (2004). *Monitoring the health of populations: Statistical principles and methods for public health surveillance*. Oxford, England and New York: Oxford University Press.

Bourdieu, P. (1984). *Distinction: A social critique of the judgement of taste*. Cambridge, MA: Harvard University Press.

Bourdieu, P., Chamboredon, J.-C., & Passerson, J.-C. (1968/1991). *The craft of sociology: Epistemological preliminaries*. Berlin and New York: Walter de Gruyter.

Brooke, G.E. (Comp.). (1926). *Code télégraphique AA* [The AA Cable Code] (2nd ed.). Singapore: C.A. Ribeiro.

Brownstein, J.S., Freifeld, C., Reis, B., & Mandl, D. (2008). Surveillance sans frontières: Internet-based emerging infectious disease intelligence and the HealthMap project. *PLOS Medicine*, 5(7): 1019–1024.

Burns, J. F. (1994, September 25). Medical experts fear refugees may spread India plague. *New York Times*, p. 18.

Bynum, W. F. (1993a). Nosology. In W.F. Bynum & R. Porter (Eds.), *Cambridge encyclopedia of the history of medicine* (pp. 335–356). London and New York: Routledge.

Bynum, W. F. (1993b). Policing hearts of darkness: Aspects of the International Sanitary Conferences. *History and Philosophy of the Life Sciences, (15)*3: 421–434.

Calain, P. (2007a). Exploring the international arena of global public health surveillance. *Health Policy and Planning*, 22(1): 2–12.

Calain, P. (2007b). From the field side of the binoculars: a different view on global public health surveillance. *Health Policy and Planning*, 22(1): 13–20.

Callon, M. (1994). Four models for the dynamics of science. In J. C. Petersen, G. E. Markel, S. Jasanoff, & T. Pinch (Eds.), *Handbook of science and technology studies* (pp. 29–63). London: Sage.

Callon, M. (2001). Actor network theory. In N. Smelser & P. Baltes (Eds.), *International Encyclopedia of the social and behavioral sciences* (pp. 62–66). Oxford, England: Pergamon.

Campos, P. (2004). *The obesity myth*. New York: Gotham Books.

Canguilhem, G. (1988). *Ideology and rationality in the history of the life sciences* (A. Goldhammer, Trans.). Cambridge, MA: MIT Press.

Cash A., & Narasimhan, V. (2000). Impediments to global surveillance of infectious diseases: Economic and social consequences of open reporting. *Bulletin of the World Health Organisation, 78*(2000): 1358–1367.

Castel, R. (1994). Problematization as a mode of reading history. In J. Goldstein (Ed.), *Foucault and the writing of history* (pp. 237–252). Oxford, England and Cambridge, MA: Blackwell.

Castellvi, M. T. C., Bagot, R. E., & Palatresi, J. V. (2001). Automatic term detection: A review of current systems. In D. Bourigault, C. Jacquemin, & M.C. L'Homme (Eds.), *Recent advances in computational terminology* (pp. 53–88). Amsterdam and Philadelphia: John Benjamins.

Centers for Disease Control and Prevention (CDC). (1994). *Addressing emerging infectious disease threats: A prevention strategy for the United States.* Atlanta, GA: U. S. Department of Health and Human Services, Public Health Service.

Centers for Disease Control and Prevention (CDC). (1998). *Preventing emerging infectious diseases: A strategy for the 21st century.* Atlanta, GA: Centers for Disease Control and Prevention.

Centers for Disease Control and Prevention (CDC). (2008). *Syndromic surveillance: An applied approach to outbreak detection.* Http://www.cdc.gov/ncphi/disss/nndss/syndromic.htm (retrieved 2009, October 18).

CDC Guidelines Working Group. (2001).Updated guidelines for evaluating public health surveillance systems. *MMWR, 50*(RR13), 1–35. Http://www.cdc.gov/mmwr/preview/mmwrhtml/rr5013a1.htm (retrieved 2009, October 6).

Cefaï, D. (2008, October). Looking (desperately?) for cultural sociology in France. Paper presented at the American Sociology Association Conference.

Cefaï, D., & Kurasawa, F. (2008). *The pragmatist turn in the French social sciences.* Unpublished book proposal.

Chateauraynaud, F., & Torny, D. (1999). *Les sombres précurseurs: Une sociologie pragmatique de l'alerte et du risque.* Paris: Éditions de L'École des Hautes Études en Sciences Sociales.

Chen, L. C., Evans, T. G., & Cash, R. A. (1999). Health as a global public good. In K. Inge, I. Grunberg, & M. A. Stein (Eds.), *Global public goods: International cooperation in the 21st century* (pp. 284–304). New York: Oxford University Press.

"China and the internet: The party, the people and the power of cyber-talk." (2006, April 27). *The Economist.* Http://www.economist.com/world/display-story.cfm?story_id=6850080, (retrieved 2009, October 18).

Chu, M. C. (2005, March). *The Global Outbreak Alert and Response Network (GOARN).* Paper presented at the International Conference on Biosafety and Biorisks. Summary by J. Nuzzo. Http://www.upmc-biosecurity.org/website/events/2005_biosafety/speakers/chu/chu.html, (retrieved 2009, October 18).

Civil Society Organizations and Global Health Governance. (2007). Http://www.wsir.pwias.ubc.ca/2007/index.php (retrieved 2009, October 18).

Coburn, D. (2000). Income inequality, social cohesion and the health status of populations: The role of neo-liberalism. *Social Science & Medicine, 51*(1): 139–146.

Coburn, D., Denny, K., Mykhalovskiy, E., McDonough, P., Robertson, A., & Love, R. (2003). Population health in Canada: A brief critique. *American Journal of Public Health, 93*(3): 392–396.

Collier, S. J., & Lakoff, A. (2006). Vital Systems Security. *ARC Working Paper, 2.* Http//www.anthropos-lab.net (retrieved 2009, January 13).

Collier, S. J., Lakoff, A., & Rabinow, P. (2004). Biosecurity: Towards an anthropology of the contemporary. *Anthropology Today, 20*(5): 3–7.

Cooper, M. (2006). Pre-empting emergence: The biological turn in the war on terror. *Theory, Culture & Society, 23*(4): 113–135.

Dato, V., Shephard, R., & Wagner, M. M. (2006). Outbreaks and investigations. In M. M. Wagner, A. W. Moore, & R. Aryel (Eds.) *Handbook of biosurveillance* (pp. 13–26). Amsterdam: Elsevier.

Davies, S. (2008) Securitizing Infectious Disease. *International Affairs, 84*(2): 295–313.

Davis, P., & Howden-Chapman, P. (1996). Translating research findings in to health policy. *Social Science and Medicine, 43*(5): 865–72.

Dean, M. (1996). Putting the technological into government. *History of the Human Sciences, 9*(3): 47–68.

Dean, M. (1999). *Governmentality: Power and rule in modern society.* London and New York: Sage.

Dean, M. (2001). Demonic societies. In T. Hansen, & F. Stepputat (Eds.), *States of imagination: Ethnographic explorations of the postcolonial state* (pp. 41–64). Durham, NC: Duke University Press.

Dean, M. (2004). *Nomos* and the politics of world order. In W. Larner & W. Walters (Eds.), *Global governmentality: Governing international spaces* (pp. 40–58). London: Routledge.

Dean, M. (2007). *Governing societies.* Berkshire and New York: Open University.

Delaporte, F. (1986). *Disease and civilization* (A. Goldhammer, Trans.). Cambridge, MA: MIT Press.

Deleuze, G. (1986/1988). *Foucault* (S. Hand, Trans.). Minneapolis, MN: University of Minnesota Press.

Deleuze, G. (1995). Postscript on control societies. *Negotiations.* (M. Joughin, Trans.) (pp. 177–182). New York: Columbia University Press.

Diamond, T. (1992). *Making gray gold: Narratives of nursing home care.* Chicago and London: University of Chicago Press.

Dillon, M. (1995). Sovereignty and governmentality: From the problematics of the "New World Order" to the ethical problematic of the world order. *Alternatives, 20*(3): 323–368.

Dodgson, R., Lee, K., & Drager, N. (2002). *Global health governance: A conceptual review.* Http://whqlibdoc.who.int/publications/2002/a85727_eng.pdf, (retrieved 2008, November 1).

Dorolle, P. (1968). Old plagues in the jet age: International aspects of present and future control of communicable diseases. *British Medical Journal, 4*(5634): 789–792.

Dowsett, G., & Couch, M. (2007). Male circumcision and HIV prevention: Is there really enough of the right kind of evidence? *Reproductive Health Matters, 15*(29): 33–44.

Dutt, A. K., Akhtar, R., & McVeigh, M. (2006). Surat plague of 1994 re-examined. *Southeast Asian Journal of Tropical Medicine and Public Health, 37*(4): 755–760.

Dybul, M. (2008, August). *Human capacity development in the US President Emergency Plan for AIDS Relief: Positive synergies between health systems and global health initiatives, non-commercial satellite (MOSAT16).* Paper presented at the XVII International AIDS Conference. Mexico: Mexico City.

Eakin, J., Robertson, A., Poland, B., Coburn, D., & Edwards, R. (1996). Towards a critical social science perspective on health promotion. *Health Promotion International, 11*(2): 157–165.

Ebright, J. R., Altantsetseg, T., & Oyungerel, R. (2003). Emerging infectious diseases in Mongolia. *Emerging Infectious Diseases, 9*(12): 1509–1515.

Emerging infectious diseases. (1993a, June). *Weekly Epidemiological Record, 25*: 186–188.

Emerging infectious diseases. (1993b, December). *Weekly Epidemiological Record,* 49: 364–367.

England, R. (2007). The dangers of disease specific programmes for developing countries. *British Medical Journal, 2007*(335): 565.

England, R. (2008). The writing is on the wall for UNAIDS. *British Medical Journal, 2008*(336): 1072.

"Epidemiological Surveillance." (1976). *International Journal of Epidemiology,* 5(1): 4–6.

Epstein, D.B. (1995). Recommendations for a regional strategy for the prevention and control of emerging infectious diseases in the Americas. *Emerging Infectious Diseases,* 1(3): 103–105.

Esposito, R. (2008). *Bios: Biopolitics and philosophy* (T. Campbell, Trans.). Minneapolis, MN: University of Minnesota Press.

Evans, R. G., Barer, M. L., & Marmor, T. R. (1994). *Why are some people healthy and others not? The determinants of health of populations.* New York: Aldine de Gruyter.

Ewald, F. (1991). Insurance and risk. In G. Burchell, C. Gordon, & P. Miller (Eds.), *The Foucault effect* (pp. 197–210). Chicago: University of Chicago Press.

Ewald, F. (2002). The return of Descartes's malicious demon: An outline of a philosophy of precaution. In T. Baker & J. Simon (Eds.), *Embracing risk: The changing culture of insurance and responsibility* (pp. 273–301). Chicago: University of Chicago Press.

Fabian, J. (2002). *Time and the other: How anthropology makes its object.* New York: Columbia.

Falk, R. (1992). *Explorations at the end of time.* Philadelphia: Temple University Press.

Fantini, B. (1993). Les organisations internationales face à l'émergence de maladies infectieuses nouvelles. *History & Philosophy of the Life Sciences,* 15: 435–457.

Farmer, P. (1999). *Infections and inequalities: The modern plagues.* Berkeley: University of California Press.

Fidler, D. (1996). Globalization, international law, and emerging infectious diseases. *Emerging Infectious Diseases,* 2(2): 77–84.

Fidler, D. (1999). *International law and infectious diseases.* Oxford, England: Oxford University Press.

Fidler, D. (2001). The globalization of public health: The first 100 years of international health diplomacy. *Bulletin of the World Health Organization,* 79(9): 842–849.

Fidler, D. (2003). Emerging trends in international law concerning global infectious disease control. *Emerging Infectious Diseases,* 9: 285–290.

Fidler, D. (2004a). Revision of the World Health Organization's International Health Regulations. *ASIL Insights.* Http://www.asil.org/insights/insigh132.htm (retrieved 2009, October 18).

Fidler, D. (2004b). *SARS, governance and the globalization of disease.* London: Palgrave Macmillan.

Fidler, D. (2005). From International Sanitary Conventions to global health security: The new International Health Regulations. *Chinese Journal of International Law,* 4(2): 325–392.

Fidler, D. (2006). Biosecurity: Friend or foe for public health governance? In A. Bashford (Ed.), *Medicine at the border: Disease, globalization and security, 1850 to the present* (pp. 196–218). Basingstoke, Hampshire, New York: Palgrave Macmillan.

Fidler, D., & Gostin, L.D. (2006). The new International Health Regulations: An historic development for international law and public health. *Journal of Law Medicine and Ethics,* 34(1): 85–94.

Fidler, D., & Gostin, L.D. (2008). *Biosecurity in the global age*. Stanford, CA: Stanford Law and Politics.

Formenty, P., Roth, C., Gonzalez-Martin, F., Grein, T., Ryan, M., Drury, P., et al. (2006). Les pathogènes émergents, la veille internationale et le Règlement sanitaire international (2005). *Médecine et Maladies Infectieuses, 36*(1): 9–15.

Foster, S. O., & Gangarosa, E. (1996). Passing the epidemiologic torch from Farr to the world: The legacy of Alexander D. Langmuir. *American Journal of Epidemiology 144*(Suppl. 8): S65–73.

Foucault, M. (1976). *The archaeology of knowledge and the discourse on language* (A. Sheridan, Trans.). New York: Harper Colophon.

Foucault, M. (1976/1978). *The history of sexuality: Vol. 1. An introduction* (R. Hurley, Trans.). New York: Pantheon.

Foucault, M. (1975/1979). *Discipline and punish*. (A. Sheridan, Trans.). New York: Vintage Books.

Foucault, M. (1986). *The history of sexuality: Vol. 2. The use of pleasure* (R. Hurley, Trans.). New York: Vintage Books

Foucault, M. (1988). On Problematization. *History of the Present* (Spring): 16–17.

Foucault, M. (1977/1994a). Entretien avec Michel Foucault. In D. Defert, F. Ewald, & J. Legrange (Eds.), *Dits et écrits, 1954–1988* (Vol. 3, pp. 140–160). Paris: Gallimard.

Foucault, M. (1980/1994b). La Poussière et le nuage. In D. Defert, F. Ewald, & J. Legrange (Eds.), *Dits et écrits, 1954–1988* (Vol. 4, pp. 10–19). Paris: Gallimard.

Foucault, M. (1980/1994c). Table ronde du 20 mai 1978. In D. Defert, F. Ewald, & J. Legrange (Eds.), *Dits et écrits, 1954–1988* (Vol. 4, pp. 20–34). Paris: Gallimard.

Foucault, M. (1994d). Titres et travaux. In D. Defert, F. Ewald, & J. Legrange (Eds.), *Dits et écrits, 1954–1988* (Vol. 1, pp. 842–846). Paris: Gallimard.

Foucault, M. (1979/1997). The politics of health in the eighteenth century. In P. Rabinow (Series Ed.) & J. Faubion (Vol. Ed.), *Power: Essential works of Foucault 1954–1984* (Vol. 3, pp. 90–107). New York: The New Press.

Foucault, M. (1998). Foucault. In P. Rabinow (Series Ed.) & J. Faubion (Vol. Ed.), *Aesthetics, method, epistemology: Essential works of Foucault 1954–1984*: (Vol. 2, pp. 459–463). New York: The New Press.

Foucault, M. (2000a). Governmentality. In P. Rabinow (Series Ed.) & J. Faubion (Vol. Ed.), *Power: Essential works of Foucault 1954–1984* (Vol. 3, pp. 201–222). New York: The New Press.

Foucault, M. (2000b). Truth and Power. In P. Rabinow (Series Ed.) & J. Faubion (Vol. Ed.), *Power: Essential works of Foucault 1954–1984* (Vol. 3, pp. 111–133). New York: The New Press.

Foucault, M. (2003). Society must be defended. In M. Foucault, *Lectures at the Collège de France, 1975–1976* (D. Macey, Trans., pp. 239–263). New York: Picador.

Foucault, M. (2007). *Sovereignty, territory, population: Lectures at the Collège de France, 1877–1978*. Houndmills, Hampshire: Palgrave Macmillan.

Franklin, S. (2000). Life itself: Global nature and the genetic imaginary. In S. Franklin, C. Lury, & J. Stacey (Eds.), *Global nature, global culture* (pp. 188–277). London: Sage.

Fraser, N. (2005). Reframing justice in a globalizing world. *New Left Review, 36*(Nov.–Dec.): 69–88.

Freifeld, C. C., Mandl, K. D., Reis, B. Y., & Brownstein, J. S. (2008, April). HealthMap: Global infectious disease Monitoring through automated classification and visualization of Internet media reports. *Journal of the American Medical Informatics Association 15*(2): 150–157.

Frenk, J. (2008, May 8–9). *Strengthening health systems: Towards new forms of global cooperation.* Plenary address, Meeting on Global Health and the United Nations. Atlanta, GA: Carter Center. Http://www.paho.org/English/D/Global-HealthandtheUN_JFKeynote.pdf, (retrieved 2009, October 18).

Frohlich, K., Corin, E., & Potvin, L. (2001). A theoretical proposal for the relationship between context and disease. *Sociology of Health and Illness, 23*(6): 776–797.

Garrett, L. (1994). *The coming plague: Newly emerging diseases in a world out of balance.* New York: Farrar, Straus and Giroux.

Garrett, L. (2007). The challenge of global health. *Foreign Affairs, 86*(1): 14–38.

Godlee, F. (1994). WHO in Crisis. *British Medical Journal, 309*: 1424–1428

Goodman, N. (1971). *International health organizations and their work.* Edinburgh and London: Churchill Livingstone.

Gostin, L. (2004a). The International Health Regulations and beyond. *The Lancet Infectious Diseases, 4*(10): 606–607.

Gostin, L. (2004b). International infectious disease law: Revision of the World Health Organization's International Health Regulations. *JAMA, 291*(21): 2623–2627.

Green, M.S., & Kaufman, Z. (2002). Surveillance for early detection and monitoring of infectious disease outbreaks associated with bioterrorism. *Israel Medical Association Journal, 4*(7): 503–506

Grein, T. W., Kamara, K. B., Rodier, G., Plant, A. J., Bovier, P., Ryan M. J., et al. (2000). Rumours of disease in the global village: Outbreak verification. *Emerging Infectious Diseases, 6* (2): 97–102.

Griffith, A., & Smith, D. (2005). *Mothering for schooling.* New York and London: Routledge.

Hardey, M. (2001). Doctor in the house: The Internet as a source of lay health knowledge and the challenge to expertise. *Sociology of Health & Illness, 21*(6): 820–835.

Hardiman, M. (2003). The revised International Health Regulations: A framework for global health security. *International Journal of Antimicrobial Agents, 21*(2): 207–211.

Hardt, M., & Negri, A. (2000). *Empire.* Cambridge, MA: Harvard University Press.

Hart, J. (2006). The Soviet biological weapons program. In M. Wheelis, L. Rózsa, & M. Dando (Eds.), *Deadly cultures: Biological weapons since 1945* (pp. 132–156). Cambridge, MA: Harvard University Press.

Harvey, D. (1989). *The condition of postmodernity: An inquiry into the origins of cultural change.* Oxford, England: Blackwell.

Hayes, M. V., & Dunn, J. R. (1998). *Population health in Canada: A systematic review.* (CPRN Study No. H-01). Ottawa, Canada: Renouf Publishing. http://www.cprn.com/documents/19187_en.pdf (retrieved 2009, January 12).

Health Gap. (2006). *GAO report on PEPFAR Prevention Programs: U.S. abstinence/being faithful-only programs produce stigma and death.* Http://www.healthgap.org/camp/pepfar_docs/HGAPPepfar0406.pdf (retrieved 2009, October 18).

Health Threats Unit at Directorate General Health and Consumer Affairs of the European Commission. (2007). MedISys (Medical Intelligence Systyem). Http://medusa.jrc.it/ (retrieved 2009, October 18).

Hedgecoe, A. (2004). *The politics of personalised medicine: Pharmacogenetics in the clinic.* Cambridge, UK: Cambridge University Press.

Hein, W., Bartsch, S., & Kohlmorgen, L. (Eds.) (2007). *Global health governance and the fight against HIV/AIDS.* Houndmills, UK: Palgrave Macmillan.

Henderson, D. A. (1976). Surveillance of smallpox. *International Journal of Epidemiology, 5*(1): 19–28.

Henderson, D. A. (1993). Surveillance systems and intergovernmental cooperation. In S. Morse (Ed.), *Emerging viruses* (pp. 283–289). New York and Oxford, England: Oxford University Press.

Henderson, D.A. (2007). Lessons learned from smallpox eradication and severe acute respiratory system outbreak. Part 1: The use of surveillance in the eradication of smallpox and poliomyelitis. In N.M. M'ikanatha, R. Lynfield, C.A. Van Beneden, & H. de Valk (Eds.), *Infectious disease surveillance* (pp. 501–510). Malden, MA: Oxford, Blackwell.

Henig, R. M. (1993). *A dancing matrix: Voyages along the viral frontier.* New York: Alfred A. Knopf.

Heymann, D. L. (2002). Infectious agents. In R. Detels, J. McEwen, R. Beaglehole, & H. Tanaka (Eds.), *Oxford textbook of public health* (pp. 171–191). Oxford, England: Oxford University Press.

Heymann, D. L. (2006). SARS and emerging infectious diseases: A challenge to place global solidarity above national sovereignty. *Annals Academy of Medicine Singapore, 35*(5): 1–4.

Heymann, D. L., Barakamfitiye, D., Szczeniowski, M., Muyembe-Tamfum, J.-J., Bele, O., & Rodier, G. (1999). Ebola hemorrhagic fever: Lessons from Kikwit, Democratic Republic of the Congo. *The Journal of Infectious Diseases, 179*(Suppl. 1): S293–S296.

Heymann, D. L., & Rodier, G. (1998). Global surveillance of communicable diseases. *Emerging Infectious Diseases, 4*(3): 362–365.

Heymann, D. L., & Rodier, G. (2004). Global surveillance, national surveillance, and SARS. *Emerging Infectious Diseases, 10*(2): 173–175.

Heymann, D. L., Rodier, G., & WHO Operational Support Team to the Global Outbreak Alert and Response Network. (2001). Hot spots in a wired world: WHO surveillance of emerging and re-emerging infectious diseases. *The Lancet Infectious Diseases, 1*: 345–353.

Hitchcock, P., Chamberlain, A., Van Wagoner, M., Inglesby, T., & O'Toole, T. (2007). Challenges to global surveillance and response to infectious disease outbreaks of international importance. *Biosecurity and Bioterrorism: Biodefense Strategy, Practice, and Science, 5*(3): 206–227.

Howard-Jones, N. (1975). *The scientific background of the International Sanitary Conferences, 1851–1938.* Geneva, Switzerland: World Health Organization.

Huber, V. (2006). The unification of the globe by disease: The International Sanitary Conferences on cholera, 1851–1894. *The Historical Journal, 49*(2): 453–476.

Hughes, J. M., & Drotman, D. P. (2008). In memoriam: Joshua Lederberg (1925–2008). *Emerging Infectious Diseases, 14* (6): 981–983. Http://www.cdc.gov/ncidod/EID/index.htm(retrieved 2009, October 18).

Hunt, A., & Wickham, G. (1994). *Foucault and law.* London: Pluto Press.

IHR News. (2007, December 11). *The WHO Quarterly Bulletin on IHR Implementation, 1.*

Inda, J. X. (Ed.). (2005). *Anthropologies of modernity.* Malden, MA: Blackwell.

Institute of Medicine (IOM). (1988). *The future of public health.* Washington, DC: National Academies Press.

Institute of Medicine (IOM). (1992). *Emerging infections: Microbial threats to health in the United States.* Washington, DC: National Academies Press.

Institute of Medicine (IOM). (2003). *Microbial threats to health: Emergence, detection, and response* (M. S. Smolinski, M. A. Hamburg, & J. Lederberg, Eds.). Washington, DC: National Academies Press.

Institute of Medicine and National Research Council. (2008). *Achieving sustainable global capacity for surveillance and response to emerging diseases of zoonotic origin* (A. Beatty, K. Scott, & P. Tsai, rapporteurs). Washington, DC: National Academies Press.

International Health Partnership. (2008). Update on the International Health Partnership and related initiatives (IHP+): Prepared for the third H8 informal meeting 22 July 2008, Washington, DC. Http://www.internationalhealthpartnership.net/pdf/IHP_Report_on_Progress_3_18_July_2008_EN_FINAL.pdf (retrieved 2009, October 18).

International Health Regulations (IHR). July 25, 1969. 764 United Nations Treaty Series 3. Http://treaties.un.org/doc/publication/unts/volume%20764/volume-764-i-10921-english.pdf (retrieved 2009, October 18).

International Health Regulations (IHR). (2005/2008). 2nd ed. Geneva, Switzerland: World Health Organization. Http://www.who.int/csr/ihr/en/ (retrieved 2009, October 18).

International Sanitary Regulations (ISR). May 25, 1951. 175 *United Nations Treaty Series* 215.

Jack, A. (2007, September 28). From symptom to system: How health aid can skew state priorities. *Financial Times.* Http://www.ft.com/cms/s/0/2318ea9c-6d60-11dc-ab19-0000779fd2ac.html (retrieved 2009, October 18).

Jackson, B. E. (2005). *Practices of knowing population health: A study in authorizing and stabilizing scientific knowledge.* Unpublished doctoral dissertation, York University—Toronto, Canada.

Kazatchkine, M. (2008, August 4). *Positive synergies between health systems and global health initiatives, non-commercial satellite (MOSAT16).* Paper presented at the XVII International AIDS Conference 2008. Mexico City, Mexico.

Keating, P., & Cambrosio, A. (2003). *Biomedical platforms: Realigning the normal and the pathological in late-twentieth-century medicine.* Cambridge, MA: MIT Press.

Kaul, I., Grunberg, I., & Stern, M. A. (Eds.). (1999). *Global public goods: International cooperation in the 21st Century.* New York: Oxford University Press.

Keane, J. (2003). *Global civil society?* Cambridge, UK: Cambridge University Press.

Kelle, A. (2007) Securitization of International Health: Implications for Global Governance and the Biological Weapons Convention, *Global Governance,* 13: 217–235.

Kickbusch, I. (2000). The development of international health policies—accountability intact? *Social Science & Medicine,* 51: 979–989.

Kickbusch, I. (2002). Influence and opportunity: Reflections on the U.S. role in global public health. *Health Affairs,* 21(6): 131–141.

Kickbusch, I. (2003a). The contribution of the World Health Organization to a new public health and health promotion. *American Journal of Public Health,* 93(3): 383–389.

Kickbusch, I. (2003b). Global health governance: Some theoretical considerations on the new political space. In K. Lee (Ed.), *Health impacts of globalization* (pp. 192–203). Houndmills, Hampshire, and New York: Palgrave Macmillan.

Kickbusch, I. (2003c). SARS: Wake-up call for a strong global health policy. *Yale Global Online.* Http://yaleglobal.yale.edu (retrieved 2009, October 18).

Kickbusch, I. (2005). Action on global health: Addressing global health governance challenges. *Public Health,* 119: 969–973.

Kickbusch, I. (2006). *Globalization, women, and health in the 21st century.* Houndmills, Basingstoke, Hampshire, and New York: Palgrave Macmillan.

Kilbourne, E. D. (1993). Afterword: A personal summary presented as a guide for discussion. In S. Morse (Ed.), *Emerging viruses* (pp. 290–295). New York and Oxford, England: Oxford University Press.

King, N. (2001). *Infectious disease in a world of goods.* Unpublished doctoral dissertation, Harvard University—Cambridge, MA.

King, N. (2002). Security, disease, commerce: Ideologies of postcolonial global health. *Social Studies of Science,* 35(5–6): 723–789.

Koenders, B. (2008, August 5) *Global financial architecture.* Panel Discussion of the Special session (TUSS01) of the XVIII International AIDS Conference. Mexico City, Mexico.

Koplan, J. (2001). CDC's strategic plan for bioterrorism preparedness and response. *Public Health Reports, 116*(Suppl. 2): 9–17.

Kraus, C. (2003, April 24). The SARS epidemic: The overview; travellers urged to avoid Toronto because of SARS. *New York Times.* http://query.nytimes.com/gst/fullpage.html?res=9902E1D71F3AF937A15757C0A9659C8B63 (retrieved 2009, October 18).

Krause, R. (1993). Foreword. In S. Morse (Ed.), *Emerging viruses* (pp. xvii–xix). New York and Oxford, England: Oxford University Press.

Krause, R. (1981). *The restless tide: The persistent challenge of the microbial world.* Washington, DC: National Foundation for Infectious Diseases.

Labonté, R. (1995). Population health and health promotion: What do they have to say to each other? *Canadian Journal of Public Health, 86*(3): 165–168.

Lakoff, A. (2006). Techniques of preparedness. In T. Monahan (Ed.), *Surveillance and Security* (pp. 265–274). New York and London: Routledge.

Lam, S. K. (1998). Emerging infectious diseases—Southeast Asia. *Emerging Infectious Diseases, 4*(92): 145–147.

Langmuir, A. D. (1963). The surveillance of communicable diseases of national importance. *The New England Journal of Medicine, 268*: 182–192.

Langmuir, A. D. (1976). William Farr: Founder of modern concepts of surveillance. *International Journal of Epidemiology, 5*: 13–18.

Larner, W., & Walters, W. (Eds.). (2004a). *Global governmentality: Governing international spaces.* London and New York: Routledge.

Larner, W., & Walters, W. (2004b). Introduction: Global governmentality. In W. Larner & W. Walters (Eds.), *Global governmentality: Governing international spaces* (pp. 1–20). London and New York: Routledge.

Latour, B. (1987). *Science in action.* Cambridge, MA: Harvard University Press.

Latour, B. (1993). *We have never been modern.* Cambridge, MA: Harvard University Press.

Last, J. M. (2001). *A dictionary of epidemiology* (4th ed.). New York: Oxford University Press.

League of Nations Health Committee. (1925). *Health organisation: Report of the Health Committee to the Sixth Assembly.* Geneva, Switzerland: League of Nations.

Learmonth, M. (2003). Making health services management research critical: A review and a suggestion. *Sociology of Health and Illness, 25*(1): 93–119.

Lederberg, J., & Shope, R.E. (1992). Preface. In J. Lederberg, R. E. Shope, & S. C. Oaks (Eds.), *Emerging infections: Microbial threats to health in the United States* (pp. v–x). Washington, DC: National Academies Press.

Lederberg, J. (1993). Viruses and humankind: Intracellular symbiosis and evolutionary competition. In S. Morse (Ed.), *Emerging viruses* (pp. 3–9). New York and Oxford: Oxford University Press.

LeDuc, J. W., Childs, J. E., Glass, G .E., & Watson, A. J. (1993). Hantaan (Korean hemorrhagic fever) and related rodent viruses. In S. Morse (Ed.), *Emerging viruses* (pp. 149–158). New York and Oxford, England: Oxford University Press.

Lee, K. (Ed.). (2003). *Health impacts of globalisation: Towards global governance.* Houndmills, Basingstoke, Hampshire (England) and New York: Palgrave Macmillan.

Lee, K., Buse, K., & Fustukian, F. (Eds). (2002). *Health policy in a globalising world.* Cambridge, UK: Cambridge University Press.

Lee, K., & Dodgson, R. (2003). Globalization and cholera: Implications for global governance. In K. Lee (Ed.), *Health impacts of globalization* (pp. 123–143). Houndmills, Hampshire (England) and New York: Palgrave Macmillan.

Lefort, C. (1986/1988). *The political forms of modern society.* Cambridge, MA: MIT Press.

Lefort, C. (1988). *Democracy and political theory* (D. Macey, Trans.). Cambridge, MA: Polity.

Leive, D. M. (1976). *International regulatory regimes: Case studies in health, meteorology, and food.* Lexington, MA: Lexington Books.

Letgers, L. J., Brink, L. H., & Takafuji, E. T. (1993). Are we prepared for a viral epidemic emergency? In S. Morse (Ed.), *Emerging viruses* (pp. 269–282). New York and Oxford, England: Oxford University Press.

Levinson R. (1998). Issues at the interface of medical sociology and public health. In G. Scambler & P. Higgs (Eds.), *Modernity, medicine and health: Medical sociology towards 2000* (pp. 66–81). London and New York: Routledge.

Lipschutz, R. (2005). Global civil society and global governmentality. In G. Baker & D. Chandler (Eds.), *Global civil society: Contested futures* (pp. 171–185). London and New York: Routledge.

Loughlin, K., & Berridge, V. (2002). *Global health governance: Historical dimensions of global governance* (Centre on Global Change & Health, Discussion Paper No. 2). London School of Hygiene & Tropical Medicine and World Health Organization's Department of Health & Development. Http:// www. who.int/entity/trade/GHG/en/index.html *(retrieved 2009, January 13).*

Lupton, D. (1994). *Moral threats and dangerous desires: AIDS in the news media.* London: Taylor & Francis.

Lupton, D. (1995). *The imperative of health: Public health and the regulated body.* London: Sage.

Luken, P., & Vaughan. S. (2006). Standardizing childrearing through housing. *Social Problems, 53*(3): 299–331.

Lyon, D. (2003). *Surveillance after September 11.* Cambridge, MA: Polity.

McInnes, C., & Lee,K. (2006). Health, security and foreign policy. *Review of International Studies, 32*(1): 5–23.

MacKellar, L. (2005). Priorities in global assistance for health, AIDS, and population. *Population and Development Review, 31*(2): 293–312.

Madoff, L. C. (2004). ProMED-mail: An early warning system for emerging diseases. *Clinical Infectious Diseases, 39*: 227–232.

Madoff, L. C., & Woodall, J. P. (2005). The Internet and the global monitoring of emerging diseases: Lessons from the first 10 years of ProMED-mail. *Archives of Medical Research, 36*: 724–730.

Mahler, H. (1966). The tuberculosis programme in the developing countries. *Bulletin of the International Union against Tuberculosis and Lung Disease, 37*: 77–82.

Manderson, L. (1995). Wireless wars in the eastern arena: Epidemiological surveillance, disease prevention and the work of the Eastern Bureau of the League of Nations Health Organisation, 1925–1942. In P. Weindling (Ed.), *International health organizations and movements, 1918–1939* (pp. 109–133). Cambridge, UK: Cambridge University Press.

Mawudeku, A., & Blench, M. (2006, August). *Global public health intelligence network.* Paper presented at the 7th Conference of the Association for Machine Translation in the Americas. Cambridge, MA. Http://www.mt-archive.info/ MTS-2005-Mawudeku.pdf (retrieved 2009, October 18).

Mawudeku, A., Lemay, R., Werker, D., Andraghetti, R. & St. John, R. (2007). The Global Public Health Intelligence Network. In N.M. M'ikanatha, R. Lynfield, C.A. Van Beneden, & H. de Valk, (Eds.), *Infectious disease surveillance* (pp. 304–317) Malden, MA: Oxford, Blackwell.

McCoy, L. (1998). Producing "what the deans know": Cost accounting and the restructuring of post-secondary education. *Human Studie, 21*(4): 395–418.

McCoy, L. (2008). Institutional ethnography and constructionism. In Holstein J. & Gubrium J. (Eds.), *Handbook of constructionist research* (pp. 701–714). New York: Guilford Press.

McNabb, S., Chungong, S., & Ryan, M. (2002). Conceptual framework of public health surveillance and action and its application in health sector reform. *BMC Public Health*, 2(2). Http://www.biomedcentral.com/1471–2458/2/2 (retrieved 2009, October 18).

Medina, M. (2003). Time management and CNN strategies (1980–2000). In A.B. Albarran & A. Arrese (Eds.), *Time and media markets* (pp. 81–95). Mahwah, NJ: Lawrence Erlbaum.

Memmi, D. (1996). *Les gardiens du corps*. Paris: Éditions de l'école des hautes études.

Merianos, A., & Peiris, M. (2005). International Health Regulations. *The Lancet*, 366: 1249–1251.

Michaud, C. (2003, October). *Development assistance for health (DAH): Recent Trends and Resource Allocation*. Unpublished paper prepared for Second WHO Consultation, Commission on Macroeconomics and Health. Geneva, Switzerland.www.who.int/macrohealth/events/health_for_poor/en/dah_trends_nov10.pdf (retrieved 2009, October 18).

M'ikanatha, N. M., Lynfield, R., Van Beneden, C. A., & de Valk, H. (Eds.). (2007). *Infectious disease surveillance*. Malden, MA: Oxford, Blackwell.

Miller, P., & Rose N. (1990). Governing economic life. *Economy and Society*, 19(12): 1–31.

Mitchell, G., & McTigue, K. (2007). The US obesity epidemic: Metaphor, method, or madness? *Social Epistemology*, 21(4): 391–423.

Moeller, S. D. (1999). *Compassion fatigue: How the media sell disease, famine, war and death*. New York and London: Routledge.

Morse, S. (1992). Epidemiologic surveillance for investigating chemical or biological warfare and for improving human health. *Politics and the Life Sciences*, 11(1): 28–29.

Morse, S. (Ed.). (1993a). *Emerging viruses*. New York and Oxford, England: Oxford University Press.

Morse, S. (1993b). Examining the origins of emerging viruses. In S. Morse (Ed.), *Emerging viruses* (pp. 10–28). New York and Oxford, England: Oxford University Press.

Morse, S. (1993c). Preface. In S. Morse (Ed.), *Emerging viruses* (pp. vii–xi). New York and Oxford, England: Oxford University Press.

Morse, S., Rosenberg, B., & Woodall, J. P. for the ProMED Steering Committee Drafting Subgroup. (1996). ProMED global monitoring of emerging diseases: Design for a demonstration program. *Health Policy*, 38: 135–153.

Murray, C., Lopez, A., & Wibulpolprasert, S. (2004). Monitoring global health: Time for new solutions. *British Medical Journal*, 329: 1096–1100.

Mykhalovskiy, E. (2003). Evidence-based medicine: Ambivalent reading and the clinical recontextualization of science. *Health: An Interdisciplinary Journal for the Social Study of Health, Illness and Medicine*, 7(3): 331–352.

Mykhalovskiy, E. (2008). Beyond decision making: Class, community organizations and the healthwork of people living with HIV/AIDS. Contributions from institutional ethnographic research. *Medical Anthropology: Cross Cultural Studies in Health and Illness*, 27(2): 136–63.

Mykhalovskiy, E., & Weir, L. (2004). The problem of evidence-based medicine: Directions for social science. *Social Science and Medicine*, 59(5): 1059–1069.

Mykhalovskiy, E. & Weir, L. (2006). The Global Public Health Intelligence Network and early warning outbreak detection: A Canadian contribution to global health. *Canadian Journal of Public Health*, 97(1, Global Health Issue): 42–44.

Mykhalovskiy, E., Armstrong, P., Armstrong, H., Bourgeault, I., Choiniere, J., Lexchin, E., Peters, S., & White, J. P. (2008). Qualitative research and the politics of knowledge in an age of evidence: The possibilities and perils of immanent critique. *Social Science and Medicine, 67*(1): 195–203.

Navarro, V. (2007). *Neoliberalism, globalization, and inequalities: Consequences for health and quality of life.* Amityville, NY: Baywood.

Negri, A. (2002). *Du retour: Abécédaire biopolitique.* Paris: Calmann-Lévy.

Nicoll, A., Jones, J., Aavitsland, P., & Giesecke, J. (2005). Proposed new International Health Regulations. *British Medical Journal, 330*: 321–322.

Ng, R. (1990). Immigrant women: The construction of a labour market category. *Canadian Journal of Women and the Law, 4*: 96–112.

Ng, R. (1995). Multiculturalism as ideology: A textual analysis. In M. Campbell & A. Manicom (Eds.), *Experience, knowledge, and ruling relations: Explorations in the social organization of knowledge* (pp. 35–48). Toronto, Canada: University of Toronto Press.

Organisation for Economic Co-operation and Development (OECD). (2008). *Measuring aid to health.* http://www.oecd.org/dataoecd/20/46/41453717.pdf (retrieved 2009, October 18).

OECD-DAC. (2008). Development Co-operation Directorate. Purpose of aid charts: Focus on aid to health. Www.oecd.org/dac/stats/health (retrieved 2009, January 12).

Office of the Auditor General of Canada. (2008). Chapter 5-Surveillance of infectious diseases—Public Health Agency of Canada. In Office of the Auditor General of Canada, *Report of the Auditor General of Canada.* Http://www.oag-bvg.gc.ca/internet/docs/aud_ch_oag_200805_05_e.pdf (retrieved 2009, October 18).

Ojakangas, M. (2006). *A philosophy of concrete life: Carl Schmitt and the political thought of late modernity.* Bern, Switzerland: Peter Lang.

O'Malley, P. (2004). *Risk, uncertainty and government.* London: Cavendish Press/Glasshouse Press.

O'Malley, P. (2005). Governing risks. In A. Sarat (Ed.), *The Blackwell companion to law and society* (pp. 292–308). Oxford, England: Blackwell.

O'Malley, P., Weir, L., & Shearing, C. (1997). Governmentality, criticism, politics. *Economy and Society, 26*(4): 501–517.

Ong, A. (2006). *Neoliberalism as exception.* Durham, NC: Duke University Press.

Ong, A., & Collier, S. J. (Eds.). (2005). *Global assemblages: Technology, politics and ethics as Anthropological problems.* Malden, MA: Oxford; Carlson, Australia: Blackwell.

Onuf, N. (2005). Media, cultural citizenship and the global public sphere. In R. Germain & M. Kenny (Eds.), *The idea of global civil society* (pp. 48–65). London and New York: Routledge.

Ooms, G., Van Damme, W., Baker, B. K., Zeitz, P., & Schrecker, T. (25 March 2008). The 'diagonal' approach to global fund financing: A cure for the broader malaise of health systems? *Globalization and health, 4*(6): doi:1186/1744–8603-4-6 (retrieved 2009, October 7).

Packard, R., Brown, P. J., Berkelman, R. L., & Frumkin, H. (2004). Introduction: Emerging Illness as Social Process. In R. Packard, P. J. Brown, R. Berkelman, & H. Frumkin (Eds.), *Emerging illnesses and society* (pp. 1–35). Baltimore and London: Johns Hopkins University Press.

Paquet, C., Coulombier, D., Kaiser, R., & Ciotti, M. (2006). Epidemic intelligence: A new framework for strengthening disease surveillance in Europe. *Eurosurveillance, 11*(12): pii=665. Http://www.eurosurveillance.org/ViewArticle.aspx?ArticleId=665, (retrieved 2009, October 7).Parascandola, M. (1998). Epidemiology: Second-rate science? *Public Health Reports, 113*(July–August): 312–20.

Pearce, N. (1996). Traditional epidemiology, modern epidemiology and public health. *American Journal of Public Health, 86*(5): 678–683.

Peters, C. J., Johnson, E. D., Jahrling, P. B., Ksiazek, T. G., Rollin, P.E., White, J., et al. (1993). Filoviruses. In S. Morse (Ed.), *Emerging viruses* (pp. 159–175). New York and Oxford, England: Oxford University Press.

Petersen, A. (2002). The new genetics and the media. In A. Petersen & R. Bunton (Eds.), *The new genetics and the public's health* (pp. 103–134). London and New York: Routledge.

Petersen, A., & Bunton, R. (1997). *Foucault, health and medicine.* London: Routledge.

Petersen, A., & Lupton, D. (1996). *The new public health: Health and self in the age of risk.* London: Sage.

Petryna, A., Lakoff, A., & Kleinman, A. (2006). *Global pharmaceuticals: ethics, markets, practices.* Durham, NC: Duke University Press.

"PEPFAR and the fight against AIDS." (2007). *The Lancet, 369*(9568): 1141. doi:10.1016/S0140–6736(07)60536–4.

PLoS Medicine Editors. (2007). How is WHO responding to global public health threats? *PLoS Medicine 4*(5): e197. doi:10.1371/journal.pmed.0040197.

Plotkin, B. J., & Kimball, A. M. (1997). Designing an international policy and legal framework for the control of emerging infectious diseases: First steps. *Emerging Infectious Diseases, 3*: 1–9.

Plotkin, B. J., Hardiman, M., González-Martin, F., & Rodier, G. (2007). Infectious disease surveillance and the International Health Regulations. In N. M. M'ikanatha, R. Lynfield, C. A. Van Beneden, & H. de Valk (Eds.), *Infectious disease surveillance* (pp.18–31). Malden, MA: Oxford, Blackwell.

Poland, B., Coburn, D., Robertson, A., Eakin, J., & Members of the Critical Social Science Group. (1998). Wealth, equity and health care: A critique of a "population health" perspective on the determinants of health. *Social Science & Medicine, 46*(7): 785–798.

Power, M. (2007). *Organized uncertainty: Designing a world of risk management.* Oxford, England and New York: Oxford University Press.

Predicting and tracking pandemics: HealthMap.org tracking H1N1 flu hot spots in real time. *Medicine & Health/Diseases.* Http://www.physorg.com/news160325542.html (retrieved 2009, October 18).

Preston, R. M. (1995). *The hot zone.* New York: Anchor Books.

Preston, R. M. (1997). *The cobra event.* New York: Ballantine.

Primrose, A. (1925). Report of the Conference on Medical Services in Canada: Chairman's Address. *Canadian Medical Association Journal, 15*(3): 244–254.

Proceedings and Recommendations of the Expert Working Group on Emerging Infectious Disease Issues: Lac Tremblant Declaration. (1994). *Canada Communicable Disease Report, 20S2* (December): 1–21.

Rabinow, P., & Rose, N. (2003). Thoughts on the concept of biopower today. Http://www.lse.ac.uk/collections/sociology/pdf/RabinowandRose-Biopower-Today03.pdf (retrieved 2009, October 18).

Raphael, D. (Ed.). (2004). *Social determinants of health: Canadian perspectives.* Toronto: Canadian Scholars' Press.

Rankin, J., & Campbell, M. (2006). *Managing to nurse: Inside Canada's health care reform.* Toronto, Canada: University of Toronto Press.

Raška, K. (1966). National and international surveillance of communicable diseases. *WHO Chronicles, 20*: 315–321.

Raška, K. (1968). Concept of epidemiological surveillance of communicable diseases, *Israel Journal of Medical Sciences, 4*(3): 402–14.

Reingold, A. (2003). If syndromic surveillance is the answer, what is the question? *Biosecurity and Bioterrorism: Biodefense Strategy, Practice, and Science, 1*(2): 77–81.

Rettie, J. (1994, September 26). Red alert in Bombay and New Delhi as plague fear shifts to more Indian cities (p. 10). *The Guardian.*

Robertson, A. (1998). Shifting discourses on health in Canada: From health promotion to population health. *Health Promotion International, 13*(2): 155–166.

Rodier, G. (2001). Confronting a world of infectious diseases. *Public Health Reports, 116*(Suppl. 2): 2–4.

Roelsgaard, E. (1974). Health regulations and international travel. *WHO Chronicle, 28*: 265–268.

Rose, N. (1999). *Powers of freedom.* Cambridge, UK: Cambridge University Press.

Rose, N. (2007). *The politics of life itself: Biomedicine, power, and subjectivity in the twenty-first century.* Princeton, NJ and Oxford, England: Princeton University Press.

Rose, N., & Miller, P. (1992). Political power beyond the state: Problematics of government. *British Journal of Sociology, 43*(2): 173–205.

Rose, N., & Novas, C. (2004). Biological citizenship. In A. Ong & S. J. Collier (Eds.), *Global assemblages: Technology, politics, and ethics as anthropological problems* (pp. 439–463). Malden, MA: Blackwell.

Rose, N., O'Malley, P., & Valverde, M. (2006). Governmentality. *Annual Review of Law and Social Science, 2*: 83–104.

Rosenberg, B. H. (1992). The politics of epidemiological surveillance, *Politics and the Life Sciences, 11*(2): 193.

Rousseau, L.-J., & Depecker, L. (1999). Nouveaux outils pour la néologie. *Réseau international de néologie et de terminologie, 20*: 2–3.

Russel, A. (2008, August). Civil society perspectives on positive synergies. Noncommercial satellite (MOSAT16), XVII International AIDS Conference 2008. Positive Synergies Between Health systems and Global Health Initiatives.

Sassen, S. (2006). *Territory, authority, rights: From medieval to global assemblages.* Princeton, NJ and Oxford, England: Princeton University Press.

Schatz, G. S. (2005). International Health Regulations. *ASIL Insight.* Http://www.asil.org/insights/2005/08/insights050802.html (retrieved 2009, October 18).

Schieber, G., Fleisherm, L., & Gottret, P. (2006). Getting real on public health financing. *Finance and Development 43*(4). Http://www.imf.org/external/pubs/ft/fandd/2006/12/schieber.htm, (retrieved 2009, October 18).

Schmitt, C. (1922/1985). *Political theology* (G. Schwab, Trans.). Cambridge, MA: MIT Press.

Schmitt, C. (1932/1996). *The concept of the political* (G. Schwab, Trans.). Chicago and London: University of Chicago.

Schmitt, C. (2006). *The nomos of the earth in the international law of Jus Publicum Europaeum* (G. L. Ulmen, Trans.). New York: Telos.

Schneider, M.-J. (2006). *Introduction to public health* (2nd ed.). Sudbury, MA: Jones and Bartlett.

Schneider, W. H. (Ed.). (2002). *Rockefeller philanthropy and modern biomedicine: International initiatives from World War I to the Cold War.* Bloomington: Indiana University Press.

Seale, C. (2002). *Media and health.* London: Sage.

Seale, C. (2003). Health and media: An overview. *Sociology of Health & Illness, 25*(6): 513–531.

Shah, G. (1997). *Public health and urban development: The plague in Surat.* New Delhi, India; Thousand Oaks/London: Sage.

Shapin, S., & Shaeffer, S. (1994). *Leviathan and the air pump.* Princeton, NJ: Princeton University Press.

Shope, R. E., & Evans, A. E. (1993). Assessing geographic and transport factors and recognition of new viruses. In S. Morse (Ed.), *Emerging viruses* (pp. 109–119). New York and Oxford, England: Oxford University Press.

Singer, B. (2004). Montesquieu, Adam Smith and the discovery of the social. *Journal of Classical Sociology*, 4(1): 31–57.

Singer, B., & Weir, L. (2006). Politics and sovereign power: Considerations on Foucault. *European Journal of Social Theory*, 9(4): 443–465.

Singer, B., & Weir, L. (2008). Sovereignty, governance and the political. *Thesis 11*, 94(August): 49–71.

Skocpol, T. (1992). *Protecting soldiers and mothers: The political origins of social policy in the United States*. Cambridge, MA: Harvard University Press.

Smith, D. (1974a). Women's perspective as a radical critique of sociology. *Sociological Inquiry* 44: 1–13.

Smith, D. (1974b). The social construction of documentary reality. *Sociological Inquiry* 44: 257–268.

Smith, D. (1987). *The everyday world as problematic: A feminist sociology*. Toronto: University of Toronto Press.

Smith, D. (1990a). *Texts, facts and femininity: Exploring the relations of ruling*. New York: Routledge.

Smith, D. (1990b). *The conceptual practices of power: A feminist sociology of knowledge*. Boston: Northeastern University Press.

Smith, D. (1999). *Writing the social: Critique, theory and investigations*. Toronto: University of Toronto Press.

Smith, D. (2005). *Institutional ethnography: A sociology for people*. Lanham, MD: AltaMira Press.

Smith, G. (1988). Policing the gay community: An inquiry into textually-mediated social relations. *International Journal of the Sociology of Law*, 16(2): 163–183.

Smith, R. (2005). *Infectious disease and risk: Lessons from SARS*. London: The Nuffield Trust.

Smith, R., Beaglehole, R., & Woodward, D. (2003). *Global public goods for health: Health economics and public health*. Oxford, England: Oxford University Press.

Sosin, D. M. (2003). Syndromic surveillance: The case for skilful investment. *Biosecurity and Bioterrorism: Biodefense Strategy, Practice, and Science*, 1(4): 247–253.

Spitler, H. (2001). Medical sociology and public health: Problems and prospects for collaboration in the new millennium. *Sociological Spectrum*, 21: 247–263.

Stabile, C. A. (1997). From the cold war to the hot zone: Nature, capitalism, and the postmodern apocalypse. *Cultural Logic: An Electronic Journal of Marxist Theory and Practice*, 1(1). Http://eserver.org/clogic/1–1/stabile.html (retrieved 2009, October 18).

Stevenson, N. (2005). Media, cultural citizenship and the global public sphere. In R. D. Germaine & M. Kenny (Eds.), *The idea of global civil society: Politics and ethics in a globalizing era* (pp. 67–83). London and New York: Routledge.

Stilberschmidt, G., Matheson, D., & Kickbusch, I. (2008, May 13). Creating a committee C of the World Health Assembly. *The Lancet, 371*: 1483–1486.

Strathern, M. (1995). The nice thing about culture is that everyone has it. In M. Strathern (Ed.), *Shifting contexts: Transformations in anthropological knowledge* (pp. 153–156). London and New York: Routledge.

Strathern, M. (1999). Regulation, substitution and possibility. In J. Edwards, S. Franklin, E. Hirsch, F. Price, & M. Strathern (Eds.), *Technologies of procreation: Kinship in the age of assisted conception* (pp. 171–202). London and New York: Routledge.

Stoto, M. A., Schonlau, M. & Mariano, L. (2004). Syndromic surveillance: Is it worth the effort? *Chance, 17*(1), 19–24.

Straus, R. (1957). The nature and status of medical sociology. *American Sociological Review, 22*: 200–204.

The surveillance of communicable diseases. (1968). *WHO Chronicle, 22*(10): 439–444.

Susser, M., & Susser, E. (1996). Choosing a future for epidemiology: I. Eras and Paradigms. *American Journal of Public Health, 86*(5): 668–673.

Thacker, S. B. (2000). Historical development. In S. Teutsch & R.E. Elliott (Eds.), *Principles and practice of public health surveillance* (pp. 1–16). Oxford, England: Oxford University Press.

Thacker, S. B., & Berkelman, R. L. (1988). Public health surveillance in the United States. *Epidemiological Reviews, 10*: 164–190.

Thacker, S. B., Goodman, R. A., & Dicker, R. C. (1990). Training and service in public health practice, 1951–90—CDC's epidemiologic intelligence service. *Public Health Reports, 105*: 599–603.

Thacker. S. B., & Gregg, M. B. (1996). Implementing the concepts of William Farr: The contributions of Alexander D. Langmuir to public health surveillance and communications. *American Journal of Epidemiology, 144* (Suppl. 8): S23–S28.

Thomas, C., & Weber, M. (2004). The politics of global health governance: Whatever happened to "Health for All by the Year 2000"? *Global Governance 10*: 187–205.

Tilson, H. & Berkowitz, B. (2006) The Public Health Enterprise. *Health Affairs, 25* (4): 900–910.

Tucker, J. B. (2005). Updating the International Health Regulations. *Biosecurity and Bioterrorism: Biodefense Strategy, Practice, and Science, 3*: 338–347.

Tulchinsky, T. H., & Varavikova, E. A. (2000). *The new public health: An introduction for the twenty-first century.* San Diego, CA: Academic Press.

Turner, B. (2003). Social capital, inequality and health: The Durkheimian revival. *Social Theory & Health, 1*(1): 4–20.

United Nations Development Programme. (1994). *Human Development Program.* New York and Oxford, England: Oxford University Press.

United States President's Emergency Plan for AIDS Relief. About PEPFAR. Http://www.pepfar.gov/about/index.htm (retrieved 2009, October 18).

UNA-USA. (1997). *Crisis and reform in United Nations' financing: A report of the UNA-USA Global Policy Project.* New York: UNA-USA Publications Department.

Uplekar, M., & Raviglione, M. (2007). The "vertical-horizontal" debates: Time for the pendulum to rest (in peace)? *Bulletin of the World Health Organization, 85*(5): 413–414.

Velimirovic, B. (1976). Do we still need international health regulations? *The Journal of Infectious Diseases, 133*(4): 478–482.

Virilio, P. (1997). *Pure war* (2nd ed.). New York: Semiotext(e).

Wagner, M. M. (2006). Introduction. In M. M. Wagner, A. W. Moore, & R. Aryel (Eds.), *Handbook of biosurveillance* (pp. 3–12). Amsterdam: Elsevier.

Wagner, M. M. et al. (2001). The emerging science of very early detection of disease outbreaks. *Journal of Public Health Management Practice 6*(6): 51–59.

Wakefield, S., & Poland, B. (2005). Family, friend or foe? Critical reflections on the relevance and role of social capital in health promotion and community development. *Social Science & Medicine, 60*(12): 2819–2832.

Wald, P. (2008). *Contagious: Cultures, carriers, and the outbreak narrative.* Durham, NC and London: Duke University Press.

Watney, S. (1997). *Policing desire: Pornography, AIDS and the media.* London: Cassell.

Wheelis, M. L. (1992). Strengthening biological weapons control through global epidemiological surveillance. *Politics and the Life Sciences, 11*(2): 179–189.

Weir, L. (1996). Recent developments in the government of pregnancy. *Economy and Society, 25*(3): 372–392.

Weir, L. (2006). *Pregnancy, risk and biopolitics: On the threshold of the living subject.* London: Routledge.

Weir, L. (2008). The concept of truth regime. *Canadian Journal of Sociology,* 33(2): 367–389.

Weir, L., & Mykhalovskiy, E. (2006). The geopolitics of global public health surveillance in the twenty-first century. In A. Bashford (Ed.), *Medicine at the border: Disease, globalization and security, 1850 to the present* (pp. 240–263). New York: Palgrave Macmillan.

Weldon, R. A. (2001). An "urban legend" of global proportion: An analysis of nonfiction accounts of the Ebola virus. *Journal of Health Communication,* 6(3): 281–294.

Whaley, F., & Mansoor, O. D. (2006). SARS Chronology. In World Health Organization, *SARS: How a Global Epidemic Was Stopped* (pp. 3–48). Geneva, Switzerland: World Health Organization.

World Health Organization (WHO). (1946). *Constitution of the World Health Organization.* 14 United Nations Treaty Series 185.

World Health Organization (WHO). (1958). *The first ten years of the World Health Organization.* Geneva, Switzerland: World Health Organization.

World Health Organization (WHO). (1968). *The second ten years of the World Health Organization.* Geneva, Switzerland: World Health Organization.

World Health Organization (WHO). (1971). *Fifth general programme of work covering a specific period (1973–1977 inclusive)* Geneva, Switzerland: World Health Organization.

World Health Organization (WHO). (1994). *Report of WHO meeting on emerging infectious diseases* (Geneva, Switzerland, April 25–26). Geneva, Switzerland: World Health Organization. Http://whqlibdoc.who.int/hq/1994/CDS_BVI_94.2.pdf (retrieved 2009, October 18).

World Health Organization (WHO). (1995). *Report of the second WHO meeting on emerging infectious diseases* (Geneva, Switzerland, January 12–13). Geneva, Switzerland: World Health Organization. Http://whqlibdoc.who.int/HQ/1995/WHO_CDS_BVI_95.2.pdf (retrieved 2009, October 18).

World Health Organization (WHO). (1996). *Emerging and other communicable disease: Strategic plan 1996–2000* (WHO/EMC/96.1). Geneva, Switzerland: World Health Organization. Http://whqlibdoc.who.int/hq/1996/WHO_EMC_96.1.pdf (retrieved 2009, October 18).

World Health Organization (WHO). (1994/1997). Plague in India: World Health Organization international plague investigation report. In G. Shah (Ed.), *Public health and urban development: The plague in Surat* (pp. 277–290, Appendix C). New Delhi, India; Thousand Oaks/London: Sage.

World Health Organization (WHO). (1998). Revision of the International Health Regulations (Progress report, July 1998). *Weekly Epidemiological Record,* 73(31): 233–239.

World Health Organization (WHO). (2002). Top ten causes of death: The ten leading causes of death by broad income group. Geneva, Switzerland: World Health Organization. Http://www.who.int/mediacentre/factsheets/fs310.pdf (retrieved 2009, October 18).

World Health Organization (WHO). (2004). Preparedness for deliberate epidemics: Programme of work for the biennium 2004–2005. *Weekly Epidemiological Record,* 12: 113–118.

World Health Organization (WHO). (2005). *Asia pacific strategy for emerging diseases* (WPR/RC56/7). Manila, Philippines: World Health Organization Regional Office for the Western Pacific Region. Http://www.wpro.who.int/NR/rdonlyres/FCEEBB9D-21BB-4A16-8530-756F99EFDB67/0/asia_pacific.pdf (retrieved 2009, October 18).

World Health Organization (WHO). (2006a). *Biorisk management: Laboratory biosecurity guidance* (WHO/CDS/EPR/2006.6). Http://www.who.int/csr/resources/publications/biosafety/WHO_CDS_EPR_2006_6/en/index.html (retrieved 2009, October 18).

World Health Organization (WHO). (2006b). Constitution of the World Health Organization. In WHO *Basic Documents* (45th ed., Supplement, December pp. 1–18). Geneva, Switzerland: World Health Organization. Http://www.who.int/entity/governance/eb/constitution/en/ (retrieved 2009, October 18).

World Health Organization (WHO). (2007). *A safer future: Global public health security in the 21st Century.* Geneva, Switzerland: World Health Organization.

World Health Organization (WHO). (2008a). *Revision process of the International Health Regulations (IHR).* Http://www.who.int/ihr/revisionprocess/revision/en/index.html (retrieved 2009, October 18).

World Health Organization (WHO). (2008b). *Frequently asked questions about the International Health Regulations (2005).* Http://www.who.int/ihr/about/faq/en/index.html (retrieved 2009, October 18).

Wilson, J. M., Polyak, M.G., Blake, J. M., & Collman, J. (2008). A heuristic indication and warning staging model for detection and assessment of biological events. *Journal of the American Medical Informatics Association 15*: 158–171.

Wilson, K., von Tigerstrom, B., & McDougall, C. (2008). Protecting global health security through the International Health Regulations: Requirements and challenges. *Canadian Medical Association Journal, 179*(1): 44–48.

Wilson, K., Mcdougall, C., Upshur, R., & the Joint Centre for Bioethics SARS Global Health Ethics Research Group. (2006). The new International Health Regulations and the federalism dilemma. *PLoS Medicine, 3*(1): 30–34.

Woodall, J. P. (1992). Preparedness is nine-tenths of prevention. *Politics and the Life Sciences, 11*(2): 194–195.

Woodall, J. P.(1997). Official versus unofficial outbreak reporting through the Internet. *International Journal of Medical Informatics, 47*: 31–34.

Woodall, J. P. (2001). Global surveillance of emerging diseases: The ProMED-mail perspective. *Cadernos de Saúde Pública, 17*(Suppl.): 147–154.

Woodall, J. P.(2005). WHO and biological weapons investigations. *The Lancet, 365*(9460): 651.

World Health Assembly. (1995a, May 12). *Communicable disease prevention and control: New emerging and re-emerging infectious diseases.* WHO Doc. WHA48.1313.

World Health Assembly. (1995b, May 12). *Revision and updating of the International Health Regulations.* WHA48.7.

World Health Assembly. (2003a, May 28). *Revision of the International Health Regulations.* WHA56.28.

World Health Assembly. (2003b, May 28). *Severe acute respiratory syndrome (SARS).* WHA56.29.

World Health Organization Maximizing Positive Synergies Collaborative Group. (2009). An assessment of interactions between global health initiatives and country health systems. *The Lancet, 373*(20 June) (9681): 2137–2169.

Wright, S. (2007). Terrorists and biological weapons: Forging the linkage in the Clinton administration. *Politics and the Life Sciences, 25*(1–2): 57–115.

Zacher, M., & Keefe, T. J. (2008). *The politics of global health governance.* New York: Palgrave Macmillan.

Index

Printed in the United States
by Baker & Taylor Publisher Services

Printed in the United States
by Baker & Taylor Publisher Services